F.II
AT ANY AGE

Praise for *Fit at Any Age*

'This eminently readable and inspiring book should galvanize everyone, young and old, into becoming more active, fitter and healthier.'

Dr Soumya Swaminathan
Chief Scientist, WHO

'If you are one of those who have come to believe that physical fitness and age are inversely related, that fitness reduces with increasing age, then here is a masterclass—*Fit at Any Age*—which busts that belief systematically.'

Amitabh Bachchan

'A good guide which shows us that there is no such thing as too late when it comes to starting your path towards fitness. Air Marshal Iyer paints a very transparent picture about how the roadmap to being a mentally and physically fit person doesn't have to be very complicated.'

Rahul Dravid
Legendary cricketer, former captain of the Indian national cricket team

'I had innumerable fitness sessions with Air Marshal Iyer, but they were a while ago. This book is my refresher course!'

Ramanathan Krishnan
A trailblazer of Indian tennis, former world no. 3 and twice Wimbledon semifinalist

'Air Marshal Iyer concluded a brilliant career at the IAF. But, to use words Atal Bihari Vajpayee made famous, the fitness fanatic in him neither tired nor retired since. What's better, he's used his immense pursuit of fitness to convince the reader that anyone can become fit at any age. It's a must-read for all, young, middle-aged or senior.'

Shekhar Gupta
Author and Editor-in-Chief and Chairman, ThePrint

FIT
AT ANY AGE
A Practitioner's Guide

Air Marshal P.V. Iyer, AVSM, VSM (Retired)

BLOOMSBURY

NEW DELHI • LONDON • OXFORD • NEW YORK • SYDNEY

BLOOMSBURY INDIA
Bloomsbury Publishing India Pvt. Ltd
Second Floor, LSC Building No. 4, DDA Complex,
Pocket C – 6 & 7, Vasant Kunj,
New Delhi 110070

BLOOMSBURY, BLOOMSBURY INDIA and the Diana logo are
trademarks of Bloomsbury Publishing Plc

First published in India 2022
This edition published 2022

Sketches in the book have been reproduced with the
kind permission of McGraw Hill. They first appeared in
Run and Discover Your Strength by Air Marshal P.V. Iyer in 1988.
Photographs for the Appendix by Indira Jayaraman
All other images © Air Marshal P.V. Iyer

Air Marshal P.V. Iyer has asserted his right under the Indian
Copyright Act to be identified as the author of this work

ISBN: PB: 978-93-94701-09-0; e-ISBN: 978-93-94701-11-3
2 4 6 8 10 9 7 5 3

Printed and bound in India Gopsons Papers Pvt. Ltd.

To find out more about our authors and books, visit
www.bloomsbury.com and sign up for our newsletters

It is strongly recommended that you consult your doctor before beginning any
exercise programme. If you engage in this exercise or exercise programme, you
agree that you do so at your own risk, are voluntarily participating in these
activities, assume all risk of injury to yourself, and agree to release and discharge
the publisher and the author from any and all claims or causes of action, known
or unknown, arising out of the contents of this book.

I dedicate this book to the fond
memory of my wife, Kalyani (Kay),
and also to the mainstay of my life,
my three children,
Mina, Indu and Parameswaran

Contents

Contents

Foreword

Air Marshal P.V. Iyer is ninety-two years 'young'. I can vouch that in his book *Fit at Any Age*, he is speaking from personal experience.

I first met Air Marshal Iyer in the early 1990s and we have remained in close touch since then. I had just retired from the international tennis circuit and was planning to start a tennis centre. Air Marshal came to know about this through the press and reached out to me. He was with the Pondicherry University at that time. After a quick meeting, we decided to join forces and he moved to Chennai.

We had acquired a 2-acre plot for the tennis centre. Air Marshal plunged into the project of developing this land with full enthusiasm right from day one and was a driving force. Our daily activities involved raising the ground, designing the tennis court and club house, planning the drainage, etc. It was all new to me and it was most useful to have him by my side. It took about eighteen months to get the courts ready for play.

In the meantime, I found out about his passion to keep fit and an early-morning run was a regular part of our routine. Since I had just got off the tennis circuit, this was a wonderful way for me to keep fit. Some of our runs would last for more than 2 hours and you certainly get to know about your companion during that kind of an activity. I realized he had extraordinary abilities.

By September 1995, our tennis centre got off the ground and he was with us till early 2001. He was the first to arrive each morning and would be jogging around the courts as all the trainees arrived. I can't think of a better inspiration for a youngster than to see Air Marshal pushing himself to such limits of physical endurance.

In 2001, Air Marshal's family moved to the US and he took leave of us and the tennis centre. While I managed to keep in touch with him, I could not fill the void left behind in the tennis centre.

Air Marshal has made use of his vast experience to put together the steps for the path to fitness, available to any person, at any age. He has taken great pains to emphasize that this path is, as he says, 'made up of small pebbles of activity, physical and mental'.

A demonstration of the author's mental alertness is this book itself, written with clarity, content, readability and humour. In the book, he suggests many methods to challenge the mind, and thus enhance its potential.

I believe that this book will increase consciousness in a large number of people regarding the importance of fitness, and turn them towards that path made of those small pebbles.

28 March 2022   **Ramesh Krishnan**
Chennai

Foreword

Having Parameswaran Iyer, the son of the author of this book, as a friend has been beneficial in several ways. However, without doubt, the biggest bonus of knowing him has been the privilege of knowing his father, Air Marshal P.V. Iyer, often affectionately referred to as the 'Running Air Marshal'. Parameswaran and I had similar starts: we both went to the same college, a few years apart, and we both joined the same service, the Indian Administrative Service (IAS). But thereafter our lives took altogether different paths, intersecting but rarely. For that reason, the good fortune and joy of meeting Iyer Uncle came my way only after four decades of knowing Parameswaran.

It was more than worth the wait! It is impressive enough that, into his nineties, he still runs 8 to 10 kilometres a day and, as you will discover in the book, has a five-days-a-week gym routine that includes pull-ups. He redefines being old and challenges the widely held notion that physical fitness is inversely related to age. Hindus believe that, of the possible 84 lakh yonis, only good karma, over many lifetimes, entitles you to human form. Iyer Uncle is a living example of how to respect this human body/form, in times when most of us spend decades abusing it.

Without doubt, Patanjali would be proud of him; he is a true yogi.

Being a true yogi is what makes Iyer Uncle such a wonderful human being: he is humble, he is great company with a fine sense of humour, he is sincere and transparent, he is a true friend to his children and their friends, and as good an example as any of bringing earnestness to both work and play. Qualities of mind and heart that his son has fully inherited; but on his son, he remains one up: unlike Parameswaran, Iyer Uncle likes his evening drink!

This book is a must-read for every woman and man, irrespective of age. As he states in the book, Air Marshal Iyer had no special athletic background when, at the age of forty-seven, he realized that we, each one of us, have the inner strength to become fit and enjoy the many benefits of a disease-free and happy life. The book describes, with many examples of his own experience, interesting anecdotes and science-based logic, simple methods to become fit. The important message that is brought out is that we can integrate fitness maintenance easily with our everyday activities, leaving sufficient time for leisure.

The book explains why mental alertness, strength training, good eating habits and the ability to laugh, especially at your own self, are all crucial to fitness and overall health. It has suggestions to help us remain alert, engaged, composed and productive, and on how to maintain our strength and ward off its decline and how to be discerning in the choice of food. Air Marshal Iyer is as fine an example as any of the importance of fitness, how it is achievable without any big upheaval in our lives and how the process is within the capacity of each one of us, irrespective of age or gender.

Having remained overweight all my life, I am perhaps the wrong person to write a foreword to this book. Yet, in some ways, I am in the Iyer Uncle camp, rarely missing my daily exercise, which now, at the age of sixty-seven, includes a 35- to 40-kilometre cycle ride at least twice a week. In spite of the weight, I do not have any real issues of high cholesterol or sugar or blood pressure. And I look forward to Iyer Uncle's company, when available, in the evening!

I hope all those who read this book enjoy it as much as I did, and learn even more than I have learnt from it.

Rajiv Mehrishi

Preface

When we are young, we tend to take our health for granted. We may play some games or pursue athletic activities, but as we grow older, most of us tend to give up physical exercise. Time passes by and we get busy with our families and career, and lo and behold, we are in our middle age. We are no longer physically as active as we used to be. We may have put on some weight.

We are still fit and can run or play games with our children. We are preoccupied with thoughts about our plans for the children and our career path, but we also start thinking about our health. This book is specifically written for those of you who are going through this phase of life, and to cheer you up by telling you how easy it is to get back to robust fitness, with renewed enthusiasm, strength and energy. You may be in your forties, fifties, sixties or even beyond. I want to persuade you, motivate you and convince you that there is so much strength in you that you can use to reclaim the vigour of your youth, irrespective of your lifestyle so far.

Generally, people tend to think of fitness as a difficult goal to achieve, involving hours and hours of strenuous workouts, visits to the gym, and such dedication that you have to sacrifice the normal pleasures of life. In this book, I have tried to throw new light on fitness, and how it can be achieved easily, without the need to sacrifice any of your interests and pursuits. I hope to convince you about the many advantages of fitness, the obvious ones and some hidden ones.

It is around the age of fifty that we sometimes tend to fall into a defeatist state of mind, a feeling that it is too late to get back to a vigorous state of health. It is important to realize that it is never late to regain your fitness. Through this book, I plan to take you through a guided tour of the path to physical and mental fitness – the two go together. And that path is easy to tread. It is paved with small pebbles consisting of easy-to-do physical and mental activities. The transformation that happened to me, and from which I have received so many benefits, is available to each one of you. So come with me on this trip to robust health. It takes just three months to become fit, and you don't have to perform any Herculean tasks to get fit. Small little steps and you are suddenly fully fit!

I am presently ninety-two years old and am an example of a person without any athletic or sports background in his youth. While serving in the Indian Air Force, at the age of forty-seven, I was confronted with a new policy brought out by the Air Force that demanded minimum age-specific physical fitness. It was a career-defining requirement, and I set out to pass the fitness test due in a couple of months. I started jogging for a few minutes every day and gradually began running for about half an hour. A sudden revelation hit me, like a bolt of lightning, that we have, each one of us, the inner strength to become fit, with all its many splendoured manifestations. I became a devotee of fitness, and my many experiments in the field of fitness have helped me to remain fit. I want to share my experience with you, and that has led me to the writing of this book.

Acknowledgements

I had just turned ninety-two in October 2021 and was living a peaceful, leisurely life, when my son, Parameswaran (Param), came on a visit to Bangalore and suggested that I write a book on fitness. His suggestions usually take the form of convincing arguments. He made the case that I have a wealth of experience in the field of fitness, and that too after a late start at the age of forty-seven. I bought his argument and thus this book came to be – and is now being unleashed on an unsuspecting public!

I am extremely thankful to Param for his guidance throughout the writing of the book.

Mina, my eldest, has been involved in every aspect of the book. Advising me on what to include and what to omit; how to present ideas in a balanced fashion; correcting typos, sometimes the syntax, formatting the text, and ensuring that my ideas are presented in an appropriate manner. She has made sure that the text does not fall into the pitfalls of repetition and helped in adding colour to the narrative. Without her active help, I would not have been able to adhere to any schedule of submitting the manuscript to the publishers.

Indu, my second daughter, has taken a keen interest in ensuring that what I wrote was accurate and science-based. She had a big influence on my suggestions and recommendations on food.

Mina and Indu have spent countless weeks collecting suitable photographs for the book, captioning them and arranging them in a chronological fashion.

My late wife, Kalyani (Kay), my inseparable partner for fifty-seven years, has been of a great beneficial influence in my life. She would have been very excited about the preparation and publishing of this book, and would have added more value to it with her enthusiasm and support. I humbly thank her for everything good that has happened to me.

I had an exciting association with the Indian Air Force for more than thirty-six years. It has shaped me and has given me a great career, meaningful friendships and a purpose in life. I salute this unique organization and wish it greater and greater glory.

My two sons-in-law, Anand and Jayaraman, have at all times been supportive of my schemes, and they have always looked after me well during my long stay at their homes. They have also been of effective assistance while I was looking for eminent people to endorse this book. My daughter-in-law, Indira, in spite of her preoccupation with her own career as a senior economist, has always been there, looking after my fitness needs, maintaining a home gym, making sure of wholesome, tasty food, putting up with my eccentricities and letting me be a happy member of her close-knit family.

During the course of writing the book, my laptop misbehaved several times. To rein it in and control its behaviour, I often sought the help of two of my grandsons, Shankar and Ashwin, and they were always ready, willing and capable of dealing with its idiosyncrasies. Shankar also helped prepare and send to the publishers all the photographs for the book, converting them into high-resolution pictures. He also took the photograph for the front cover of this book, my doing a pull-up in the local park.

It gives me great pleasure to thank my granddaughters, Akila, Janaki and Tara, and my grandsons, Shankar, Ashwin and Venkat, for the love that they have always showered on me. There is no greater happiness for a person than to have the comfort of the affection of the younger generation. I am indeed blessed. And what is more, the spouses of these children, Sneha, Kamini, Ashwin (senior) and Ashwath, are equally affectionate towards me and have become part and parcel of my immediate family.

My three great-grandchildren, Aarav, Vara and Anika, are the joy of my life, radiating sheer happiness, mirth and fun. A few more of these joyful babies are due, and hopefully, I can write about them in another book.

It is my good fortune to have the friendship of Ramesh Krishnan, the tennis legend. It was graceful of him to write a foreword to this book with great warmth. I value my close association with Ramesh. I am grateful to Rajiv Mehrishi, former comptroller and auditor general of India, for writing a foreword in his inimitable style.

I have been very lucky to have received generous endorsements for this book from eminent personalities like Amitabh Bachchan, Ramanathan Krishnan, Dr Soumya Swaminathan, Rahul Dravid and Shekhar Gupta. My grateful thanks to them. Air Chief Marshal B.S. Dhanoa, former Air Force Chief, has always encouraged me and I am thankful to him for his support.

Many thanks to Krishan Chopra, editor-in-chief, Bloomsbury India, for his encouragement and to Paul Vinay Kumar, publisher, with whom I have interacted regularly throughout the period of writing, editing and finalizing the book. I am also thankful to Meenakshi Singh, head, marketing and publicity, for chalking out a plan to promote the book. I am truly grateful to Bloomsbury for placing their confidence in me, in my advanced age, as capable of delivering a pertinent and opportune manuscript for publication.

I am extremely grateful to Air Marshal Manavendra Singh, PVSM, AVSM, VrC, VSM, ADC, AOC-in-C Training Command, IAF, Bangalore, for all the help he has provided in launching the book, and for agreeing to preside over the book release function.

ONE

Fit at Any Age
(And Remain Fit into Your Nineties)

Ronald Reagan became President of the United States at the age of sixty-nine. When he announced his desire to run for re-election at the age of seventy-three, his opponent was fifty-six-year-old Walter Mondale. During one of the presidential debates before the election, the moderator asked Reagan, 'Mr President, you are seventy-three years old. Will you be able to bear the burden of the presidency at your age?'

To this Reagan replied, 'I will not make my age an issue in this election. I will not, for political purposes, exploit the youth and inexperience of my opponent.'

Everyone laughed and Reagan secured his second term in a landslide win. Anecdote apart, there is a big chunk of truth in what Reagan said. Wisdom and common sense mature with age. But a concerted effort is needed to remain healthy and fit as we age, a process that usually kicks in after we hit the age of sixty.

Anyone Can Be Fit, at Any Age

In this chapter, I will explain how you can continue to live a healthy life even as you grow old. It does not matter whether you are sixty, seventy or even older; it does not matter what lifestyle you have followed till now; it does not matter whether you drink alcohol or are a teetotaller; it does not matter whether you are fat or slim; it does not even matter if you have ever worked out in a gym or not! I am offering you a chance to lead a healthy lifestyle into your 'golden years'. And I will give you reasons for making such a statement without even knowing anything about you.

When we are young, we hardly think about old age. If at all the topic of old age comes up, we are so busy with our affairs that we do not pay much attention to it. I got married when I was just short of twenty-four years. My wife, Kalyani, was a few months younger. Once, while travelling by train, we met a stranger. He was into palmistry and offered to study our palms. He predicted a generally happy life and said that we would lead healthy lives till our sixties. Past sixty years of age, we could face some health issues. I remember being very happy with his prediction, as being sixty years of age seemed far, far away. Ill health never entered our thoughts as we went on to live our lives. We eventually entered our sixties and beyond, and mortality was never thought about. This is true for all of us. Whoever thinks about death? We all think it is something that happens to other people! We would like to live on till eternity.

As We Age, We Value Our Lives More

The older we get, the more we value our lives. In my eighties, I had to once consult an ear, nose and throat doctor for a slight nosebleed. I wanted to be reassured that there was nothing seriously wrong with me. The doctor did not suggest any test and instead of doing a detailed examination, he said philosophically, 'Sir, you are eighty years old now. You have lived a happy and successful life. Your children are well settled. So, there is no need to worry about your health now. Be relaxed and accept whatever comes along.'

The doctor completely missed the point. I did not go to him for compassionate advice, but to be cured if I was suffering from any ailment and be reassured that there was nothing seriously wrong with my health. Though I got rid of the nosebleed soon, the incident made me think about people's approach to illness and longevity. Generally, people want to live, no matter how old they are. We have all read about people who at the end stage of cancer have spent a quarter of a million dollars on experimental medicines hoping to prolong their lives by a few more months.

A Far-Reaching Assurance

I want to tell my readers that whatever your present age, whether you are in your fifties, sixties or more, you can have a healthy life. Your quality of life can be excellent, and you can enjoy your life and have exciting new experiences. You may be wondering how I can give such an assurance without knowing anything about you. Well, it is based on my experience, science and logic, and here are the reasons for my assurance.

Reason 1: Take It from a Ninety-Two-Year-Old

Let me cite my example. I was born on 30 October 1929. As you may have already calculated, I am ninety-two years old. Every morning I run 8 kilometres. In my youth, I was neither athletic nor into outdoor activities. It was only when I turned forty-seven that I started taking an interest in health and fitness. At that time, I was in the Indian Air Force and the then air chief introduced a policy that required all Air Force personnel to undergo a physical fitness test once a year. One of the tests required the personnel to run a mile (1.6 kilometres) in a certain number of minutes, depending on age. As I was forty-seven, I had to run a mile in less than 7 minutes. As I started practising for the test, it became fun to get up in the morning and go for a run. Within a few weeks, I could run comfortably at a fairly good pace. On the day of the test, I ran a mile within 7 minutes, and now, at the age of ninety-two, I run 8 or 9 kilometres a day and work out in the gym five days a week. To date, I have run 1,20,000 kilometres and can even do five to six pull-ups on a horizontal bar. Life has taught me that a person can become fit at any age and remain so well into their nineties. This applies to both men and women in equal measure. If you are middle-aged, it is not the time to take things easy, but to explore new things and achieve new goals. However, to enjoy your middle-aged life to the fullest, you need to be fit, and this book tells you how to be fit by following simple activities.

Reason 2: The Science of It

According to science, your health today is dependent on what you have been doing during the last three months. For example, you used to exercise regularly and were super fit but had to discontinue your fitness regime because of an injury or illness. If you were unable to follow a fitness schedule for three months, you are almost no different from a person who has never exercised. You will have to start from the beginning to build back your fitness. We have known acquaintances who became bedridden because of a fracture. In the absence of any physical activity, their limbs became atrophic and weak. To make their limbs stronger again, they had to undergo physiotherapy. Hence, activity is essential to life.

Luckily, when you enter into an exercise programme, you will become fit within three months. You will be able to compare yourself with any individual who exercises regularly. This is true for both men and women and a person of any age. If you start living a healthy life, you can be assured that the vestiges of your earlier lifestyle will not come in the way of acquiring robust health. You will be among the fittest of your peers. But to become fit, you need to devote a certain amount of time to exercise. Fitness training needs to become a part of your daily life. You can start an exercise programme at any age. So if you have decided to become fit and enjoy all the benefits of being fit, this book will guide you.

Here I want to caution the reader that you should not confuse fitness with bulging muscles and a six-pack abdomen. Fit people come in many forms and shapes. They are short, tall, thin or fat (but not obese). Some long-distance runners look half-starved. In long-distance-running circles, if you look well-fed, you have not been training! Fitness, to a large extent, is a function of the health of your heart. If your heart is efficient, every cell in your body gets a continuous supply of oxygen-rich blood. This blood nourishes the cell and the cell functions well, doing whatever job it is assigned to do, whether in the brain, kidney, liver or any other organ in the body. So, when I talk of fitness, do not expect a beautiful musculature, which is the general concept of a fit person. Rather, look for what that person can do, how much physical load he or she can take and how much stress she or he can endure. It may not necessarily be visible outwardly but you know it when you have reached it.

If you follow the guidelines given in this book, which are based on my experience over several decades devoted to fitness, and on science and logic, you are bound to become and remain fit. And there is no dispute that the fitter you are, the better your quality of life, and the lengthier your lifespan. Subsequent chapters will give you a full insight into the concept of fitness and how to achieve it. But, to become and remain fit, it is important to follow the advice given in this book regarding the lifestyle that you need to adopt from now onward. Fitness does not come by wishing alone, it needs the determination to work towards it. But remember, you do not need superhuman efforts to be fit – just normal, reasonable activities, which will be explained in detail in Chapter 3.

Reason 3

Human life expectancy is increasing all over the world. Modern medicine, advances in diagnostics, treatment and physiotherapy ensure that you have an excellent chance of recovery from an illness. In general, it is the nature of the human body to recover from illness. And if you do not delay in consulting a doctor, the chances of full recovery are even better.

Reason 4

This is an important reason. You, dear reader, have got hold of this book. It shows that you are curious enough to think about the way you are approaching your life. That is a great start. I plan to show you how exciting life is going to be. And if you follow the simple guidelines outlined in this book, you are bound to live a healthy life.

In addition to the logical reasons for being healthy and fit, which I have outlined in this book, it is important to appreciate and understand that getting old is a natural process. Old age is not a calamity or something to be worried about but is designed by evolution to enable us to pass through an enjoyable period of life that is full of new experiences, activities and achievements. Ageing is the unfolding of the magical phase of our lives when we use our knowledge and experiences to sail through the ocean of opportunities and promises. Think of old age as a period of serenity, free from the rat race of life. It is the time to enjoy your worth, your family, your friends, and whatever you are working at, to cultivate hobbies, follow your passion, travel and pursue your own special thing.

But to take advantage of your senior citizenship, you need to be healthy and this book is meant to help you become and remain fit. Whatever your age may be, to be physically and mentally fit, you need to stop telling yourself 'I am too old to exercise'.

My Surprising Discovery

When I was forty-seven years old, I made a surprising discovery. I found that the human body is a marvellous creation, capable of taking any amount of physical and mental abuse, absorbing any amount of exertion and coming up rugged and robust. That is the nature of the human body. It can endure any amount of physical hardship and come out stronger. Physically, the human body is supreme in the animal kingdom. You may think that this is an exaggeration, but let us look at it objectively. The American author George Leonard discusses an imaginary athletic contest between a man and certain animals in his book *The Ultimate Athlete*. My consideration below is based on that contest.

Let us suppose that we hold a competition among certain animals like a lion, an elephant, a horse, a cheetah, a monkey and a shark. Let us further assume that they all take part in a heptathlon race (it is a race normally held

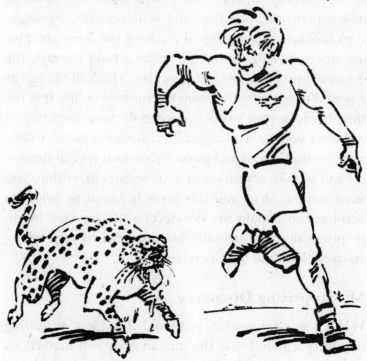

In all-round athletic ability,
no animal can match the human being.

among females where each of them participates in seven different races, including running, jumping, swimming, etc., and the woman who collects the highest points, after competing in all the seven events, is declared the winner). Let us now suppose that a woman competes with all these animals. A cheetah would easily beat her in a sprint event, as would an elephant in a throwing event like shot put, a shark would beat her in swimming and a monkey would excel in gymnastics. But overall, the woman would score the highest. She would beat all the animals in a high jump competition except the monkey, she will be better than them in swimming except the shark, she will outdo most of them in acrobatics except the monkey and she would remain unbeaten if long-distance running is included.

The Human Being: The Supreme Athlete

Human beings are supreme long-distance runners. No other animal can run long distances like us. Even a horse for all its running ability has to come to a stop after several kilometres, but the human being can carry on for several days without stopping, as has been demonstrated by many ultramarathon runners. Human beings are endowed with a large number of sweat glands, which enables them to endure the excess heat generated during prolonged physical activity. When we run, a large amount of heat is generated that needs to be cooled if we wish to continue running. Our sweat glands do this job. Animals like the cheetah, with superior speed, can only run for a minute or two by which time they have generated so much heat that they have to come to an abrupt stop. If they are unable to capture their prey in that period, they have to rest and try again. But this is not so in the case of a human being. Australia's indigenous people have a unique method of capturing kangaroos. They follow the animal, which will initially hop away out of reach. But Aboriginal Australians patiently follow them, sometimes for several days, until the poor animals can no longer stand, let alone run. The animal can then just be picked up from where it fell.

Long-Livers Come in Many Forms

A human being alone is the supreme athlete. Mahatma Gandhi had said that a human being's life is 120 years. It is another matter that he or she is struck down by violence; otherwise, they could have lived long. So can each one of us. 'Long-livers' come in all forms. Their lifestyles vary. Their food habits are different. There is a joke about a group of journalists visiting one Peter Longfellow, who was celebrating his hundredth birthday. When they asked Peter the secret of his long life, he said he led a disciplined life, abstained from alcohol and cigarettes, avoided late nights, took limited food and exercised regularly. While Peter was telling the journalists about his lifestyle, a loud sound of merrymaking came from an apartment above. When asked about it, Peter said, 'Oh, that is my elder brother, Paul. He is celebrating his one hundred and fifth birthday today. He loves his wine, loves parties and dances through the night!'

Each of Us Has Great Genes

We get our genes from our prehistoric ancestors; the men and women who lived millions of years ago. These

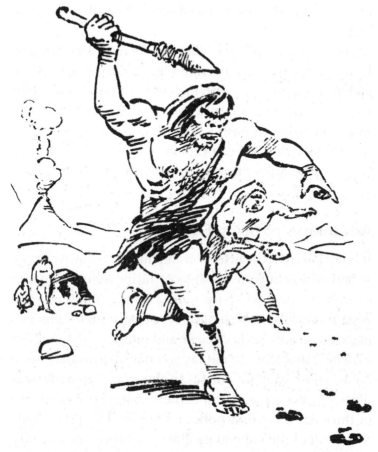

The extraordinary strength of our prehistoric ancestors
continues to exist in each one of us.

people had to lead a tough life; they depended on their
physical ability for survival. They had to run to escape
from danger, gather food and survive natural disasters.
Because of such a lifestyle, they developed strong hearts
and lungs. The genes of these ancestors are in our bodies,
in our heart, lungs and other organs. Despite the millions
of years that have gone by, these are the genes that we are
made of. Though often we are unaware of what we can

do, we can carry out extraordinary physical and mental feats.

In my previous book, *Run and Discover Your Strength*, I said that if you take up running, you can discover that you have got great strength in your body, which you never knew existed. Often, we are surprised to find that we were able to accomplish a Herculean physical task – and do it quite easily. We can exploit our inner, undiscovered strengths by attempting to do new things, both mental and physical.

Advantages of Being Fit

It is obvious that the fitter you are, the better you function. Whether it is in your workplace, during leisure activities or at home, you will have more energy, enthusiasm and zest. You will be able to navigate through minor illnesses like cold, headache, body ache and indigestion that affect us. These problems do not lay you flat whereas they often harass those who are not fit. In the case of more serious illnesses, you often get an early warning, a grace of two or three days. You may notice a sluggishness in your body as a result of the impending illness and then you can take corrective action before the disease manifests itself in all its severity. The remedy, in many cases, may be to avoid intense physical activity till the infection goes away. You also naturally have the option to consult your doctor well in time. The feeling of being superbly fit is something unique. Insurance companies in western countries are offering discounts of up to 20 per cent of the premium on life insurance policies for those who exercise. To qualify, you must certify that you exercise regularly and also undergo a physical test. If you follow the advice given in the subsequent chapters, you will be so fit that you will have no problem passing your physical examination. Marathon runners qualify automatically. Now, insurance companies employ hard-headed businessmen and women. They depend on facts and figures. So, if they part with money (in this case, in the form of a reduced premium), it is because they have statistical evidence that fitness prolongs life. You can draw your conclusions from this.

As a fit person, an additional advantage you have is an increased amount of immunity in your body, which helps you ward off illness. It will surprise you when you observe that you do not tend to fall ill. Your level of fitness has a built-in mechanism to fight infections and other maladies before they can make you sick.

Aerobics

Dr Kenneth Cooper is a pioneer in the field of fitness. A mere lack of illness, he points out, is not the same thing as being fit. He is at present ninety-one years old. He is the author of the famous book *Aerobics*. Published in 1968, *Aerobics* became an instant bestseller. In the book, Dr Cooper argues that genuine fitness can only be achieved by activities that make you consume oxygen in large quantities. The human body needs a continuous supply of oxygen to burn glycogen and produce energy to survive and for the organs to properly function. Our body gets its glycogen supply from the food we eat. Oxygen, needed to burn glycogen, is derived from the air that we breathe. The important point to remember is that though glycogen can be stored in the body (in the muscles and the liver), oxygen has to be continuously supplied in sufficient quantities through the lung–heart–blood vessels route. Oxygen cannot be stored in the body. When extra oxygen is required by the body – for example when carrying heavy weights or climbing up the stairs, or even when you are emotionally upset – your lung–heart–blood vessels system may not be able to cope with the extra need, causing a strain on your body. The theory of aerobics postulates that we can develop our capacity to deliver oxygen to our cells, even at highly increased rates, if we train the oxygen delivery system of our bodies. This then is the basic theory of genuine fitness. And this is what we will discuss in the following chapters.

Let me conclude this chapter by pointing out the great benefits of being fit. There are many books and publications that bring out the importance of exercise in keeping one fit. The latest research on exercise, published in medical journals like *The Lancet*, reaffirms the importance of exercise in being fit. Research points out that lack of exercise is a positive contributing factor to illness and curtailment of lifespan. More on that in subsequent chapters.

In ancient India, many great practitioners mastered the Indian system of medicine known as Ayurveda or the science of life. Vagbhata was one of those great scholars and writers. In one of his treatises, he wrote about the importance of exercise, which encapsulates all that needs to be said about the benefits of exercise.

Deeptagni, karma samarthyam, laghavam, dukhasahishnata, Vichitra Ghana gatratvam, vyayamaatupajayate

Roughly translated from Sanskrit, this means exercise confers an excellent digestive system, skill in performing various tasks, a light-hearted approach towards life, the capacity to bear sorrow and an astonishing body structure contributing to a strong body and mind. The benefits of exercise thus cannot be overstated.

As you start exercising regularly, you will notice certain changes that occur in your body. Many of these changes are measurable. Your heart will beat a little slower. The normal adult human heart beats at the rate of seventy-two a minute. As you start exercising, your heart rate will become slower. Into eight weeks of your exercise programme, the heart rate may become sixty-five beats a minute. Do not be surprised if it reduces further, to sixty or even fifty beats a minute after another two or three months. This is an indication that your heart has become stronger and it can perform its main function of pumping blood with more ease and less effort. This is typical of an athlete or an individual with good aerobic fitness.

Your body will show other measurable signs. You will lose weight, especially if you do not eat extra food and maintain the same eating habits that you followed before starting the exercise programme. We all know losing a few kilos of weight is good for our health. You would lose inches from your waist, and you may need to alter your existing clothes; it may be an expensive exercise but worth it. There will be other changes too that may not be measurable, but visible. You will sleep better, you will feel fresh throughout the day, you will be more energetic and you will not get tired easily. Your digestion will improve, your self-esteem will go up, you will become more confident and your personality will get a boost. For example, a woman after a 15-minute jog would have a flushed face, revealing an attractive complexion, the like of which one may not get from applying any amount of make-up. Exercise does unique things to our body and mind.

We can do astonishing things at any age. William Shatner, who played the role of Captain Kirk in *Star Trek*, flew into space on a rocket ship at the age of ninety. At the age of fifty-six, I ran 270 kilometres, from Agra to New Delhi, with a group of young men and women. Age is no bar to expressing yourself physically and mentally.

Let us get fit!

TWO

What Is Fitness and Why You Need It?

We use the term fitness very often in our daily lives. Broadly we know what it means, but when we discuss fitness at length and how to achieve it, we need to be clear about what it means. Does fitness mean having a muscular body? Is it something that bodybuilders aspire to have? Does being fit mean having a six-pack? Are we planning to run a marathon? Are we aiming to lift heavy weights? So what exactly do we mean when we say that we need to be fit?

I would say fitness is the ability to lead a healthy life. It is the ability to carry out physical and mental activities that we are called upon to do, including the pursuit of our work and other interests, and which may demand energy, strength and enthusiasm.

Being fit involves the ability to be ready for any emergency, physical or emotional, that we may be called upon to deal with. It may be a task demanding physical activity like running for some time or carrying a heavy object for some distance; it could also be emotional strength like being resilient to mental shock. All of us have had to face such situations at some point or the other in our lives. To be able to successfully execute such tasks and not get unduly strained, we need to have a robust body and mind. Let me give you a few examples from my experience.

An Unexpected Emergency

In 1988, my wife and I lived in Faridabad. One day we went to the Army Golf Course in Dhaula Kuan, Delhi, to meet my son Param and join him in a game of golf. He and I usually partnered together and played against other twosomes. After the game, we said goodbye to Param and drove back home. Five to six hundred metres from home, the car started malfunctioning and after a few yards, it came to an abrupt halt. It was dark and the area was known to be generally unsafe. With hardly any passers-by or traffic, seeking help was out of the question. Despite being an expert in car maintenance, I couldn't get the car running. With no other option left, I was forced to push it home. Luckily it was a Maruti 800. My wife steered the wheel, while I pushed the car. I don't know whether you have ever pushed a car by yourself, but I can vouch that it takes some effort. And it didn't help that I'd played bad golf in the evening!

All the lung power I had gained by running and the muscle strength I had built in the gym over the years came to my rescue. After about 20 minutes, with two or three brief halts for rest, we reached home. I did not suffer any major discomfort and a few pegs of rum helped me put the incident behind me! What I wish to emphasize is that it pays to build strength. I was fifty-nine years old at that time. Today, at the age of ninety-two, as I jog for more than 2 hours every morning and train in my home gym six days a week, I thank those hundreds of workout sessions for giving me the strength to be able to absorb the training and deal with unexpected emergencies.

Dimensions of My Training

Let me offer a glimpse of the types of training that I have undergone during my decades of experimenting with fitness, which gives me the stamina and strength to absorb the hard work. There has never been a day that I haven't run. If I was travelling on a long-distance train, I would get

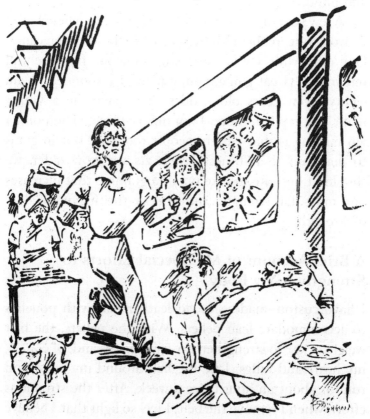

Some people will run anywhere, even on a railway platform, during a train halt, in order not to miss even one day of training!

down at a station where the train was scheduled to stop for 20 minutes and jog up and down the railway station for 15 minutes. And if the train was relatively empty, I would run in the restricted space of the compartment itself. I have run in ships, in hospitals, on mountains and in valleys. I have run on the banks of St Laurent, in Montreal, Quebec, and I have run in the snake-infested forests of Wayanad, Kerala. The diversity of places adds fun and variety to your run, enriching your body and mind.

A few years ago, I was in Washington DC. There I used to work out in the YMCA gym in Bethesda, Maryland. One day, while I was exercising, someone from behind remarked, 'Great going, young man.' I responded, 'I am eighty-seven years old – does that make me a young man?' He replied, 'Sure, I am ninety-three!' The point I am making is that elderly people too work out in gyms to maintain their fitness levels. As we grow older, we shouldn't hesitate to take up a programme that increases our muscular strength and checks the inevitable loss of strength.

A Brief Account of My Special Efforts to Strengthen My Body

I have custom-made a broad leather belt with pouches to accommodate lead pellets. With the pellets, the belt weighs 5 kg. To strengthen my leg muscles and, of course, my heart and lungs, I tie the belt around my waist and run for about an hour twice a week. After the strenuous effort, when I remove the belt, I feel so light that I believe I can actually fly.

In 1981, I was stationed at the Kanpur Air Force Base. There the banks of the Ganga were dotted with sand dunes, each about 4.5 metres high. I would run to the top of a dune, jog down and then run to and up the next dune, thus covering all the dunes. This I did twice a week for 1 hour. This regime helped me further strengthen my body. A few months later, when I took part in the First Asian Veteran Athletic Meet in Singapore, I won the gold medal in the 5,000-metre running race, leading from start to finish. I was fifty-two years old at the time and was competing against athletes from Japan, Indonesia, Malaysia, China and other countries.

The Agra to Delhi Run

Training makes us fit and enables us to carry out difficult tasks. In 1985, to celebrate the Air Force anniversary, which falls on 8 October, I organized an ultra-long-distance run, of 270 kilometres, from Agra to Delhi. About 300 young people, mostly from the armed forces, but also from other walks of life, took part in what was essentially a community run and not a race. Notable participants were a former Olympic athlete, Ranjit Bhatia; an Oxford Blue runner, Dev Lahiri; and a young marathon runner, Asha Agarwal. The gruelling run was completed by about a hundred runners, with the rest dropping off on the way. I too completed the run and handed over the Air Force flag to the then air chief marshal, Denis La Fontaine, at the Palam Air Force Parade Ground in Delhi.

As I aim to help you achieve the fitness that can be gained at any age, I feel we should discuss the various facets of fitness.

1. **Aerobic fitness (cardiovascular fitness):** This is the most important part of fitness; our very lives depend on this form of fitness. Throughout our lives, every cell in our body needs oxygen continuously. Some cells, like brain cells, need more oxygen than other cells. Cells need more oxygen when they are active than they do when they are at rest; for example, the cells of the leg need more oxygen when we are running than when we are at rest. We can get by with a weak hand but cannot survive without aerobic fitness, which ensures we have a strong heart, efficient lungs and a robust system of blood vessels.

2. **Muscular fitness:** We need strong muscles to carry out the hundreds of activities that we are expected to perform, both voluntary (like walking, carrying weights and climbing) and involuntary (like respiration and digestion). They also are engaged in maintaining the integrity of the body and protecting vital organs.

3. **Flexibility:** Flexibility plays a significant role in our fitness because it contributes to the economy of effort in all the physical activities that we do. We need to be physically flexible to avoid injuries.

4. **Speed:** Every day we encounter events when we need to move quickly. For example, to pick up a child when she is about to fall or to save ourselves or someone else from imminent danger.

5. **Mental stability:** Mental stability is an essential part of our fitness. We need to have a sound mind in order to be aware of everything around us, to be creative, to enjoy our lives in all their aspects, to base our actions on logic and to give meaning to our existence.

More about Aerobic Fitness

Aerobic fitness is our capacity to supply oxygen to the body for all its needs, and for this our heart, lungs and blood vessels need to function well. Oxygen from the lungs is taken to all parts of the body by the blood, which is pumped by the heart. Our ability to carry out all bodily and mental functions is determined by our aerobic fitness and therefore our very existence depends on it. We must achieve this form of fitness as it is a decisive, indispensable, life-or-death requisite for our well-being. Aerobic fitness ensures that our heart, lungs and blood vessels function well. The network of blood vessels is referred to as the vascular system, thus the term 'cardiovascular'. We can train our hearts to be strong and efficient as it is one of the few organs over which we can exercise some measure of control. When we exercise or work hard physically, our heart also works hard. When we rest, it beats slowly. The lungs work in close conjunction with the heart in what is known as the pulmonary system. When the heart beats faster, the lungs too heave faster and take in larger and larger quantities of oxygen-rich air.

Our Unique Ability

There is hardly any literature in medicine or fitness-related science that discusses the control we can exercise over some of our organs. So let us indulge in some original thinking about human biology. We can strengthen our minds and many parts of our bodies through some form of exercise or mental effort. For example, we can exercise our limbs, work out in the gym and strengthen the body. We can run or do exercises that make the heart beat fast, thus strengthening it. We can exercise our

minds by studying a variety of subjects: when we learn
musical instruments, languages, painting or sculpting, it
enriches our minds. As you must have deduced, while
we can directly influence many aspects of our physical
and mental health, we cannot directly influence the
functioning of our vital organs like the liver, the kidneys
and the endocrine glands. These organs perform critical
roles in our well-being and any malfunction in any of
them will affect our life quality. All we can do is ensure
that the heart beats efficiently to supply the organs with
oxygen-enriched blood that they constantly need. And
we can achieve this by keeping our cardiovascular system
functioning well.

But how do we keep the cardiovascular system
strong? By making the heart beat faster and stronger. It
may sound counter-intuitive that to become stronger, the
heart needs to work harder, but that is the truth. And that
is within our control. When we use our limbs and move
them faster and for a longer period, they demand more
and more oxygen. To supply this additional oxygen, the
heart needs to beat faster and harder. The legs, having the
biggest muscles in the body, demand more oxygen and
are the key to making the heart beat faster and stronger.
There we have it – the simple but eternally true fact. We
move our limbs, especially the legs, to work the heart
harder, to strengthen the heart. The lungs, working in
harmony with the heart, also become more efficient. The
blood vessels become more and more amenable to the
smooth flow of blood.

Avoid Blockage of Arteries

There is a rider to the above conclusion. The blood vessels
are susceptible to damage by the formation of adhesive

substances like plaques (consisting of cholesterol, among other things), which effectively reduce their diameter. This condition, in medical parlance, is known as atherosclerosis. It affects every human being, in some measure. This, in turn, affects the smooth flow of blood. If this kind of damage occurs in the coronary artery, it might obstruct the blood flowing to the heart muscles, which may cause a heart attack. The consensus of the medical fraternity is that exercise reduces the build-up of plaque in the blood vessels. And as an enthusiast of fitness and a runner of many decades, it is my firm belief that regular running significantly reduces the potential blockage of blood vessels.

As an anecdotal justification for my confidence, I would like to quote here the example of Clarence DeMar, a famous American marathon runner. He was popularly known as Mr Marathon. When he died at an old age, an autopsy was performed on his body.

The findings of the autopsy were published in the *New England Journal of Medicine* in 1961. Among other things, the results showed that DeMar's coronary arteries were two to three times the normal size. This, of course, does not lead us to any scientific conclusion regarding the benefits of regular running. But anecdotal examples do boost our confidence in the efficacy of running in preventing atherosclerosis.

The Initial Steps in Starting a Fitness Programme

Seek Medical Advice

If you have decided to follow an exercise regime, you need to assess your present fitness level. Consult a doctor if you have any concerns about your present state of health. I may add here that doctors generally are a conservative lot. If you are middle-aged, the doctor might advise you to follow a moderate exercise regime. He might discourage you from running or may not agree to carry out a treadmill test on you. Whenever I visit a doctor, I inform him or her about the kind of training I have been following. The doctor then assesses my physical condition based on this. Otherwise, if the doctor checks my pulse rate and finds it to be forty-eight beats a minute, he or she might immediately advise hospitalization! They would not know that because of the training, my resting pulse often goes down to forty or even thirty-eight. Björn Borg had a resting pulse of thirty-six. It is natural for top athletes to have a low pulse rate. So do consult a doctor before you start an exercise programme, and ensure that you do not have any ailments that could potentially debar you from attempting vigorous physical activities.

With the above caution about consulting doctors, I must add that we should seek medical advice when we have any health issues. The best advice I have had regarding fitness is that we should consult a doctor whenever we feel ill or have doubts about any health issues. One mistake we often make is to ignore warning signs about our bodies. Headache, pain in any part of the body, lack of appetite, difficulty in sleeping, the occurrence of skin lesions and many other symptoms need to be checked by a doctor. All of them are curable or treatable. More than 90 per cent of our illnesses are curable, especially when diagnosed early. So my first advice on your journey to fitness is to attend to any health issues that you may have noticed. In addition, if you are over thirty-five years, or if you have any medical problems like high blood pressure, obesity, previous history of heart disease, history of heart ailment among close relatives (parents, brothers or sisters), diabetes, or if you smoke, you should have a medical check-up before you start a new fitness programme. The check-up should include a stress cardiogram (that is, an electrocardiogram, or ECG, after strenuous exercise or a treadmill test).

Assess Your Present Fitness Level

Once you are assured about your health, it is time to self-assess your physical condition. How strong are you or your muscles? What is the extent to which you can make your limbs work? Can you walk long distances? Can you run? If so, how fast and for how long? Each of us has evolved uniquely and what we are today is the sum total of how we have spent our lives. We should be realistic in our self-assessment. Overconfidence may lead to injuries whereas underconfidence will prevent you from achieving your potential. Consider your capabilities in basic activities: these are walking, jogging, running, climbing, cycling and swimming. While any form of sport is good for physical and mental health, in this chapter we will discuss the route to aerobic fitness. This is a specialized form of fitness. To achieve this type of fitness, continuously engage the heart and lungs, without a break, for at least 20 minutes. Sporadic working of the heart and lungs and resting them in between, as happens when we play games like tennis, badminton, football or hockey, will not help us achieve the desired results.

Over a few weeks, assess yourself while you work out. You don't need to try every form of exercise. Find your favourite exercise and increase the distance or time of workout during, say, two weeks. Do not increase the time of the exercise abruptly. Increase your workout time by 15 minutes every three weeks. If you find that you get unduly tired during or after your workout, cut back immediately. You are not trying to become fit overnight. Three to six months is the time that you have to give yourself on your road to becoming fit. Your assessment of your present state of fitness should lead you to decide what exercise you prefer to do and how much of it you could do in a week.

Road to Fitness

Once you have cleared the first two steps (health check and self-assessment), you are ready to begin your journey towards becoming fit. The road to fitness is straightforward. Start by choosing your preferred and convenient form of workout. If you have chosen running, read Chapter 3, which has a complete guide on how to get fit by running. Remember, you can start a running training programme at any age. I took up running when I was forty-seven years old. Running has been my fitness mantra. As I have said elsewhere, I have logged more than 1,20,000 kilometres of running since I took it up. I still jog at least 8 kilometres every day, seven days a week.

Do Not Worry

If you have neglected your fitness, have not been exercising regularly, are obese or do not have access to open air, do not worry. Once you start a regular excise programme, your fitness level will keep on increasing and your earlier lifestyle will not come in the way of your future fitness. You will find that within three months of starting a fitness programme, you have become as fit as anyone else.

Many of us don't pay much attention to our physical fitness when we are young; in fact, we take our fitness for granted. We begin to think about our health only when we approach fifty or sixty years. That is also the time when the body throws up hints of frailty. A noticeable decrease in strength is one symptom. It is estimated that our strength begins to reduce at the rate of 10 per cent per decade from the age of thirty. Things that we could do effortlessly earlier seem to be difficult now. Lifting a child is no longer child's play. We begin to notice our declining strength, speed and flexibility during our daily activities. Memory sometimes plays tricks with us. We often accept these shortcomings as part and parcel of growing old, but we have to act decisively to check and arrest the decline. Once you make up your mind to act towards this goal, it is easy to remain fit for the rest of your lives. And if you remain fit, chances are that you will live longer.

The Way Forward

When we don't stay idle for long, when we move about, when we employ our mind in various challenging tasks, we are on our way to fitness. Our ancestors were hunter-gatherers and forever on the move. Though the human DNA is programmed to move around constantly, we have become sedentary. The human body thrives on mental and physical activities. When we employ our body to do physical activity, it becomes stronger. When we employ our mind on constructive thought, it becomes creative. If we spend a lot of time daily without being physically active, our body begins to deteriorate. Similarly, if we don't challenge our mind with thoughts and ideas, it becomes unproductive. In short, we flourish with activity and rust with lethargy. In subsequent chapters, I shall propose a way of life that will make you fit and keep you fit for the rest of your lives. You don't need to go out of your way to make Herculean efforts in becoming fit. You need not run at all; there are other exercises that you can comfortably do which will make you fit without drastically changing your existing lifestyle. Today is the first day of the rest of your life. Start working on making that future healthy and rewarding. Start becoming fit!

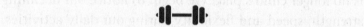

THREE

Running Your Way to Fitness

The purpose of this book is twofold. The first, discussed in Chapter 1, is to assure readers that it is possible to become fit at any age, irrespective of their past lifestyle. The second is to encourage everyone, young and old, to adopt habits that boost fitness. Let us discuss the second objective in more detail. We should encourage our children to take up games and sports, especially outdoor activities, from early childhood. A boy or girl, moulded in this fashion, will become a healthy adult and will be naturally inclined to maintain an active lifestyle. Exercise will become a central part of their life. My grandchildren also are fitness conscious and run regularly. Two of them, Tara and Venkat, are top athletes and have represented India in tennis. Though my great-grandchildren are still toddlers, I do keep an eye on their activities!

In this chapter, I will show you how to set up a running regimen. The advice applies to all, whether seeking to become fit in middle age or beginning a fitness journey when young.

Even though the advice is specific to running, the principles apply to other forms of exercise as well. In the next chapter, I will discuss the measures required to be taken for a specific exercise.

You Can Start a Running Programme at Any Age

As I have mentioned in the previous chapters, anyone at any age can take up a running programme. Apart from my example, many others started running in their eighties and nineties. For instance, Fauja Singh, who is 110 years old and lives in Britain, took up running in his nineties. He has run many marathons (42.195 kilometres), including one after he was a hundred years old! It is not just men, many women in their fifties, sixties and seventies too run regularly. My daughters, Mina (sixty-seven) and

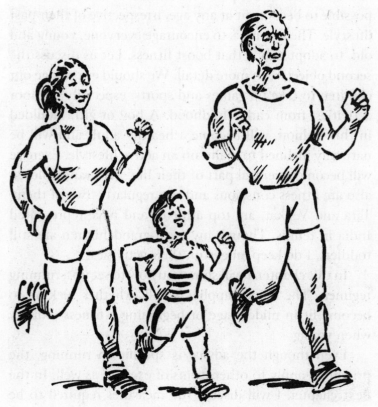

Everyone needs fitness: man, woman and child.

Indira (sixty-five), exercise regularly and often take part in 10-kilometre races. Param has been running regularly since his college days. Now at sixty-two years, he runs at least three or four times a week. His wife, Indira, also runs and works out regularly. My passion for fitness has rubbed off on my children and their families.

I have been part of the veteran athletic movement in India and know of many men and women who run and keep fit even in their old age. Running seems to come naturally to younger people. The young need to remember to maintain a regular running schedule and not to overdo things; maintain a record of daily workouts and balance exercise, academics, rest and recreation.

Running is a simple activity, and everyone knows how to run. It does not need any specialized skills as in the case of golf or tennis. However, for the novice runner, certain guidance is necessary, especially about how far, how fast and for how long.

You may not enjoy the run on your first day or even during the first few days and weeks. But stick with it and after a few days, you will gradually start enjoying the sessions. Of course, you may be a rare case who takes to running from the first day, or again, you may be a not-so-rare case who cannot cope with the regimen of daily running. But everyone starts enjoying the activity eventually after a few weeks.

Your body does not care when you run. It is only interested in the fact that you run regularly. Some, like me, prefer to run in the morning. Early morning is a pleasant time to run as it is not too hot. After completing the session, you can attend to your day's work, knowing that you are ahead of the game. Others like to run in the evenings as getting up early is torture for them. Evening runs also have advantages as the body is warm and active then. An evening run may also promote a feeling of pleasant tiredness, making it easy to sleep well. While running on an empty stomach is perfectly all right, you should never run immediately after a meal. A gap of at least 2 hours should be there between having a meal and running.

Where to Run?

When I took up running, my initial attempts were not notable or rewarding. I lived in an apartment in Green Park, Delhi, and on the first day went to the terrace to jog. My next-door neighbour had a dog who ran up to its part of the terrace. With just a small wall separating us, it started barking loudly without a pause. All the neighbours came up to investigate. The dog's owner suggested that I should just walk and not run on the terrace. Dogs, he said, don't like people doing strange things. I realized that there was no future in running on the terrace and the next day I started running on the roads. Of course, there are dogs on the road too, but by and large, they leave you alone. So, keeping a wary eye on dogs and other hazards, I embarked on my running journey.

It does not matter where you run. Choose a nearby field or other convenient spots. Some people like to run in a restricted place or on a circular track. Others prefer to go on a trail or track and enjoy the scenery. If you have a river or stream not too far away from home, you may enjoy running on its banks. Or there may be a small hillock or other scenic places. Use available space. Changing your running venue periodically is also a good idea.

Warm-Up

The human body does not respond efficiently to sudden activity. The concerned muscles and tendons need to be brought into action gradually. Animals follow this principle instinctively. Before setting forth on its affairs, a cat stretches luxuriously after it wakes up. Choose your warm-up exercises. Warm-up is done to warm up your muscles and increase the heart rate gradually, and not suddenly. For 5 minutes, do bending and stretching exercises for all the major muscle groups of the body. Start with trunk bending exercises, forward, sideways and back. Then without bending the knee, bend down and touch your toes about a dozen times. Remember your heart is also a muscle and should be brought into activity gradually. A brisk walk for a minute or two will do the trick.

On my first day of running, I had set forth on a quick run without engaging in any warming-up exercises. After about 2 minutes, I experienced an uncomfortable feeling in the chest and was forced to stop. After resting for a few minutes I felt better, but I learned my lesson. Never start any exercise programme without doing a proper warm-up. After you are warmed up, you should jog. Your aim should be to jog continuously for anything between 1 minute and 5 minutes. Following the jog, walk briskly for a minute or two and again break into a jog. The first day's workout consists of jogging followed by walking and again jogging, and so on. As soon as you feel out of breath, start walking fast. When you feel that you can jog again, do so. Alternate between jogging and walking for about 15 minutes. During the workout, if you experience any pain in the chest, you should discontinue the run and seek medical advice. You should, however, ignore minor aches and pains.

Running Speed

Let us move on to running speed. In the initial days, you should restrict yourself to jogging. Try to jog at a speed at which you feel comfortable. You should not get out of breath. Younger and fitter people may want to start at a fast speed. They may do so, but it is far better to defer running fast to a later period. Any injury suffered during the early days of your running is bound to put your schedule back and dampen your enthusiasm. Another reason to treat speed with caution is that running fast is a demanding task. It is well known among runners that it is the pace that tires you and not the distance. In the initial days of the programme, you have to put 'miles in the bank' and build a sound foundation before trying to play with speed. No doubt it is exhilarating to run fast and hard, and every runner should do at least some of his or her running at a fast pace, but that must come later, certainly not during the initial six weeks of running. As it is, you are putting your body under sufficient stress by running. You don't want to tax it further at this stage. One good method of finding out whether you are running too fast is the talk test. You should be able to carry on a conversation with a fellow runner or an imaginary fellow runner if you prefer to run alone. But make sure that no passers-by are watching you talking to yourself for they might think you are a prime candidate for the lunatic asylum! If you are too short of breath to converse, cut down your speed.

Running at a faster pace will enable you to complete your workout faster and your heart would beat faster. But you must remember that speed is not the key. I am not able to run fast now because of acute osteoarthritis. Instead, I jog slowly and complete a kilometre in 10 minutes. That is ample to keep me fit at my age. It will be different for you. Take stock of your present level of fitness and any problems you might experience while exercising. Run at a speed you are comfortable in.

Young people will find the suggested 10 minutes of activity fairly easy, though there may be some who will be surprised to see that they cannot jog at a stretch even for 5 minutes. Older people should run well within their capacity and should have some energy to spare. The walk between the jogs should be brisk and is very much a part of the workout. It helps to keep the heartbeat at a higher level, without letting it fall too much. Don't attempt any heroics and run for the whole workout; jog–walk–jog is the recipe. It does not matter at this stage how many minutes you jog and how many minutes you walk. At the end of the workout, don't stop abruptly, but keep walking slowly for about another 5 minutes. When you were running, the blood in your body was circulating at a fast rate, mainly due to your heart pumping faster and, by the pumping effect of the muscles of your legs. If you stop the activity suddenly, the pumping effect of the leg muscles is cut off and blood tends to pool at the lower extremities. In a severe case, the blood pressure might drop due to insufficient venous return to the heart. This is why one shouldn't stop running suddenly. After you have walked for about 5 minutes, you should repeat the warm-up exercises that you performed at the start of the run; they are now the cool-down exercises. These exercises will relax the muscles and lessen the chances of sore muscles and limbs. Never neglect these warm-up and cool-down exercises. If you have to skip either one due to lack of time, it is better to skip the warm-up before the run, but never the cool-down.

Acclimatization to Heat and Humidity

If you happen to be in a hot and humid region, you need to take extra care to get acclimatized to the weather. Slip into the exercise programme gradually. Even super-fit athletes get into trouble if they attempt their peak performance in hot and humid conditions without first acclimatizing themselves to the weather condition over several days. Weather conditions do not respect an individual's athleticism.

Several years ago, I saw the effect of oppressive heat on a world-class athlete in Chennai. In 1998, Boris Becker had come to Chennai to take part in an International Tennis Federation (ITF) tournament in April. He lost in the second round. His opponent in the second round was G. Solves, not a fancied player. It was the weather that was Becker's nemesis.

Acclimatization to Altitude

Another thing you need to worry about is altitude. If you plan to run or do some strenuous exercises in a hilly, high-altitude place, you need to be extremely careful. I learned my lesson in Shimla, where I had gone on a visit when I was about fifty years old. By then I had become a regular runner and did not miss a single day of running. Soon after arriving in Shimla, I set out on my usual run and ran for about 45 minutes. To my surprise, my chest started paining and it struck me that I was in a high-altitude place. Luckily for me, I got over the discomfort. I had to ease into my running training over the next few days, to run comfortably.

I used this hard-earned lesson when I took part in an important marathon race held in Bangalore in 1984. The National Veterans' Marathon was an important event that was taking place in Bangalore, which is 900 metres above sea level. I thought it was better to get acclimatized to the change in altitude and so put in some high-altitude running. Param was sub divisional officer (SDO) Dehradun at that time and I went to Dehradun and stayed with him for ten days. I would take a bus to Mussoorie (altitude 2,000 metres) every morning, run there for about 2 hours and return to Dehradun. From Dehradun, I flew directly to Bangalore for the race. Several runners had assembled, including Mr Natarajan, a very fine runner from Bombay. I enquired from Mr Natarajan whether he had been training in Bangalore for a few days. He said that he had arrived that morning from Bombay. As the starter's gun went off, Mr Natarajan shot off at his usual fast clip and the others, including myself, tried to hang on as best as we could. We had to run around Ulsoor Lake fourteen times, a lap of about 3 kilometres each circuit. At one stage, Mr Natarajan was almost 1 kilometre ahead of me. But slowly he got tired and I caught up with him on the tenth circuit. As I overtook him, I saw he could hardly jog. It was a lack of sufficient oxygen that had hit him, which in a long race like the marathon, will affect you badly. I am happy to add that I won that marathon race comfortably and the first runner-up was a good 400 metres behind me.

Breathing

A few words about breathing during the run. In the olden days, coaches used to advise runners not to breathe through the mouth but to breathe in and out only through the nose. This is impractical. It may be all right in the initial stages of your running when you are running at a slow pace and for a short period. But as you progress and start running faster and for longer durations, you won't get far if you breathe only through your nose. So open your mouth and gulp in all the air that you need. Never stuff your mouth with a handkerchief as I have seen runners in India do in long-distance races. You need plenty of oxygen and you won't get enough through your nose.

Once you have got through your first day's running, it is important to make it a regular habit. The first few weeks are the most crucial period, because this will determine whether you have entered the path towards fitness or not. It is a make-or-break period. In my case, I had the motivation to run a mile in under 7 minutes because that was the only way I could get a 'Fit' entry in my Air Force file for my next fitness test. An 'Unfit' entry would have affected my career. You have an even more important motivation: to be fit for life. So stick to your resolve and get through the initial few weeks of running. After a couple of months, you will start enjoying your newfound enthusiasm for running. It is during this period that many aspiring runners stop. This is especially applicable for runners above the age of fifty. While there may be many convincing arguments to give up – like your legs are aching, you feel tired throughout the day, you can't go to sleep, you don't have the time or there doesn't seem to be any tangible benefit from running – this is the period when you have to exert your willpower, the same willpower that made you start running in the first place.

I have nudged a few people to take up running. Colonel Padsalgikar, my bridge partner, was stationed with me in the Nagpur Air Force Headquarters of Maintenance Command. A charming person, he had many funny anecdotes to recount from his career in the army. I got him to start jogging with me every morning. He had the stamina to run for about 30 minutes. His only problem was a nagging pain in his right heel. He would run through the pain with a grimace. Luckily, the doctor diagnosed the problem: all it required was an insertion of an orthotic device on the sole of the right shoe. We continued to jog happily thereafter.

A few years later, after I had retired, I was living in Pondicherry, working as the Director of Sports at Pondicherry University. I had a young friend, Dr Mohan Kumar, in the neighbourhood. He was in his thirties and I encouraged him to run with me. Though his work schedule was demanding and he often had to attend to emergencies, he kept up at least four or five days of running.

After five years of living in Pondicherry, I moved to Chennai, where I took up the job of an administrator-cum-coach in the Krishnan Tennis Centre. Ramanathan Krishnan and Ramesh Krishnan, the two tennis legends of India, had started the coaching centre. Every morning, before the morning training sessions, Ramesh would run with me for an hour. On the weekly off days, he would invite me to the Madras Club in Adyar where we would run 20 kilometres along the river Adyar amid scenic surroundings. Occasionally, we would go to the Madras Cricket Club (MCC) in Chepauk and run around the cricket field, along the outer edge of the ground. Ramesh would run for an hour or so, then branch off for his tennis. I, on the other hand, would continue my run for another hour with a small tea break. I was sixty-six years old at that time and very fit. Much later, when I was in my eighties, Ramesh and I again met in Chennai and would run six days a week on Marina Beach. Anand Rengaswamy, the owner of Maris Hotel in Chennai, was an excellent runner and joined us in these runs. We would start from the Madras Lighthouse, run up to the Napier Bridge and run back, a distance of 6.5 kilometres. We would typically finish the run in just less than an hour. Anand and Ramesh would disperse and I would continue to run for another hour before returning home.

It takes at least six weeks of running for its benefits to show up. To quit then would be disastrous, after all the hard work that you have put in. As you continue to run, you will notice that the running becomes easier, more enjoyable and something you look forward to.

After a week of running, you can extend your workout by 2 or 3 minutes. The activity, however, continues to be the same: jog–walk–jog. Thus, every week, increase your workout time by a few minutes until you can do it for 20 minutes. Some people can reach this stage within three to four weeks while others may take a full six weeks to be able to work out for 20 minutes. It does not matter. Make progress according to your capacity, but make sure that you do progress. You should remember that the initial warm-up before the run and the final cool-down after the run are in addition to the 20 minutes of the main workout. If you apply yourself to the task, you will notice that you can jog for increasingly longer periods and the need to walk between the jogging sessions becomes progressively less. By the end of six weeks, many of you may be able to jog continuously for the full 20 minutes. But this is in no way a requirement. People who are not so young or are overweight or have no athletic background may not be able to jog continuously for more than a few minutes at a time even after six weeks. So be it. When I started running at the age of forty-seven, it took me about a month to run continuously for 10 minutes. Women generally make faster progress than men because they have more inbuilt stamina.

When you reach the stage where you can run continuously for 10 to 12 minutes, you have hit a landmark. You have become a miler! Most people can run a mile in 12 minutes. This is no mean achievement. You can try it out with your friends. Invite them for a run with you. Without some training, very few people can run continuously for 10 to 12 minutes. In the Air Force, as in other services, we had two or three fitness sessions a week in the evenings. We assemble and do fitness drills, play outdoor games and exercise for a while. In 1970, I was stationed in Chandigarh and was commanding an Air Force unit. During one of our evening physical training sessions, we decided to run and assess how long we could run at a stretch. Our group comprised twenty people and the average age was around forty years. Being the commanding officer, I had to decide which drills to perform. I told the assembled men to run at whatever speed they wanted and see how long they could run continuously. In those days, I was not into any fitness training. I took off at the speed of 7 minutes a mile and was surprised when I came to a grinding halt after only a minute or so. I could not summon up enough air to be able to continue. I was in distress. If we are not running regularly, it is not easy to run for several minutes. Most members in the group stopped running after a few brief minutes. Perhaps four or five continued for another minute or two. But all came to a stop after 5 minutes. Unless we attempt it, we cannot estimate the level of fitness required to run for 10 or 12 minutes.

Keep a Journal

Now you have reached the level of fitness required to run for 12 minutes. You are part of a select group of people who can run a mile. From now on, your progress as a runner should be more enjoyable. During this period of six weeks, you should maintain a journal and record the number of minutes you run each day, where you run and how you feel during and after the run. This is a very valuable record as it will help you see what kind of runs made you feel tired and what combination of running days and rest days worked best for you. If you ever decide to take part in races, your journal will be a reliable guide in planning your training.

You must also note in your journal your pulse rate, which should be measured every morning as you get up. The best method to count your pulse is to take a reading of the pulse for 15 seconds and multiply the figure by 4. The best place to feel the pulse is at your wrist, directly below the thumb. Over time, your morning pulse will give you an excellent indication of the improvement in your fitness.

A man's pulse at rest is about seventy-two beats a minute. For a woman, it is about seventy-eight beats a minute. As you run regularly, your resting pulse rate decreases. This would be noticeable by the end of six weeks of running. For some, it might reduce by as much as fifteen beats a minute. For others, it might reduce by only seven or eight beats a minute. But reduce it will. Your record in the journal will bear testimony to this. The significance of a lower pulse rate is that the heart can perform its normal functions with less effort. For instance, if your resting pulse has reduced from seventy-two to sixty at the end of six weeks, it means your heart is now beating 12 times less a minute or 17,280 times less a day, and carrying out all its functions with less effort. Imagine the tremendous amount of reserve strength that it has built up. Not only has it become more efficient but also has more time to rest in between the beats.

I have kept a journal ever since I started running. One journal a year, I now have forty-five journals. Though storing them is a challenge, they come in handy at times. For example, if I am injured after a workout, I refer back and check when I had a similar injury in the past, what kind of run caused that injury and what I did to get over it.

Amount of Time Devoted to Running Training

So far, I have made no mention of the time that you need to devote to your running routine. This is a highly subjective matter. We as human beings are built so differently. Some may thrive on a large amount of running, while others may want to end the running session as quickly as possible. It is, therefore, impossible to lay down any hard and fast rule. Do what is convenient and comfortable for you. There is no point in tiring yourself by overtraining. During the initial months of my running, Param and I used to run along our regular route, covering a distance of 3 kilometres. But one particular day, Param suggested, at the end of 1.5 kilometres, that we run for a total of 6 kilometres. It is a big jump, from 3 kilometres to 6 kilometres. But we did run those 6 kilometres that day. As we returned home, we were pretty exhausted. But I would not recommend this to anyone. A sudden increase in speed or mileage is not a good idea, and any increase in intensity should be gradual. To derive full benefit from your fitness regime, a minimum of 5 hours of running a week should be your goal. An occasional entry of 'Rest Day' in your running journal is a good thing. Only, that entry should not occur too often. I jog every day, without any rest days. It suits my body. During the last five years, there might perhaps have been five or six days that I might have missed out on jogging.

You may think it crazy, but I have run under circumstances when running should be the last thing on one's mind. In 1981, my two daughters were getting married within three days of each other. The family had assembled at Air Force Station Avadi, some 30 kilometres from Chennai. It was convenient for us and it was not difficult to commute to Chennai every morning for the pre-wedding and actual wedding formalities. I would get up at 3 a.m., finish my run by 5 a.m. and get ready by 6 a.m. to start the trip to Chennai. On one of those days, while running on a rocky and rugged field at 3.30 a.m., I almost trampled on a snake. I learned my lesson that if one has to run at unusual hours, one has to choose a well-lit place.

But each to his own. The make-up of each body is so unique that we cannot set down the amount of exercise a person needs, at what intensity and at what regularity. You have to experiment and decide for yourself. In doing so, you will find it very useful if you maintain an exercise log.

When you have worked out regularly for about three months, you will notice unmistakable and noticeable improvements in various aspects of fitness. Apart from a reduction in resting heart rate, you will see a reduction in your weight, especially if you are not consuming extra food. Your energy level would have increased and so too your enthusiasm for doing whatever you do. Regularity in training is also important. You should run at least five times a week to maintain your fitness. The immense benefit of your regularity will manifest itself in many noticeable ways. If you feel like it, increase your running mileage. But it should be done gradually and not more than 10 per cent a month.

Fitness cannot be stored; it has to be earned every week by working out. Fitness is not like money in the bank, which can be kept till you need that money. You can withdraw the money whenever you want. If you have not worked out for several weeks for whatever reason – travel, sickness, etc. – you will notice that you have lost a great deal of your fitness. Then you will have to begin all over again to get your fitness level back.

In concluding this chapter, let me say that fitness is by itself a great thing to have. But it need not be an end in itself. Fitness is also required to achieve your goals and your ambitions and to speed your way to where you are heading. In short, to enhance the quality of life.

Running is one of many options to earn fitness. I will deal with other options in the next chapter. But running is an interesting option for many reasons. It gets the work done fast, certainly faster than walking. It is exhilarating. Your metabolic rate remains high throughout the day and helps you to lose or maintain your weight. Lastly, running helps you to discover the ruggedness in you.

FOUR

Many Pathways to Fitness

When You Approach Middle Age

To spur us on to continue physical activities and to retain our enthusiasm to remain fit, it is useful to remind ourselves about what Father Time can do to our body and mind if we do not proactively engage in an active lifestyle. Many studies have been conducted by the World Health Organization, the Indian Council of Medical Research and the Centres for Disease Control and Prevention in the USA that highlight the crucial role played by physical exercise in warding off the adverse effects advance age plays on our body. I have analysed many of these studies and for convenience, present the results in a tabulated form.

Age (in years)	40	50	60	70	80
Extent of Muscular Strength Available (%)	80	70	60	50	40
Speed (%)	70	60	50	40	30
Flexibility (%)	60	50	40	30	20
Aerobic Capacity (%)	90	80	70	60	50

Let me explain the table for an easy understanding of what we can expect as we grow older.

Muscular Strength

Muscular strength starts declining once we reach forty, and only half of our strength remains by the time we become seventy.

Speed

We become slow as we age and our speed reduces by about 10 per cent every decade. In our sixties, we can generate only half the speed that we had when we were young.

Flexibility

As we grow older, we become less flexible. When we reach fifty, most of our joints become stiff and this affects the way we can exert our limbs to carry out various tasks. It also makes us susceptible to injury.

Aerobic Fitness

Deterioration in the pumping capacity of the heart along with the narrowing of arteries (due to a condition called atherosclerosis) adversely affects our aerobic fitness, which is, if you remember, the main form of fitness. Though aerobic fitness does not deteriorate fast, a significant amount is lost in our seventies.

Weight Gain

From the age of forty, we begin to gain weight and simultaneously lose muscle strength. By the time we approach seventy or eighty, we would have lost half of our muscle strength and gained, on average, 20 kg of weight. This condition can be described as obesity, which is a pathological condition in itself, leading to diseases like diabetes, cancer and other cardiovascular diseases.

There Is Hope for Us

Despite all the above dire tidings, there is hope for all of us. If we start an exercise programme and make it a regular habit, we can delay, to a considerable extent, the onset of the above-mentioned harmful events to our well-being. You can start such a rehabilitative and constructive plan at any age, be it fifties, sixties, seventies or even eighties. I have given my example often enough in this book. It will bear repeating once more. Today, at the age of ninety-two, every morning I thank God for another wonderful day that has been offered to me and thank my efforts over the last five decades. The long runs (sometimes over 32 kilometres), the marathons, the hours spent in gyms and my devotion to fitness have helped me lead a healthy and fruitful life. I am thankful for being able to devote several hours a day to fitness, as well as to go about pursuing other interests, including of course writing this book!

In Chapter 1, I mentioned that as we become older we become more aware of the pleasures that we can enjoy and are desirous of prolonging our lives. This desire can easily be fulfilled if we make up our minds to exercise regularly. When we are young, working out is almost effortless, but it is a precious gift that you can give yourself when you need it later in life.

Let us now see what other alternative methods are available to us to become fit.

Many Pathways to Fitness

Running, as outlined in the previous chapter, is just one method of becoming fit. There are other ways of reaching the same goal. Walking, climbing, swimming, cycling, aerobic dancing and working out on a treadmill are all efficient ways to achieve robust health. In this chapter, I shall outline guidelines on how to set about adopting alternative routes to the goal.

The central theme when employing any method for becoming fit is the same. Depending on the activity engaged in, organs and muscles demand blood at a certain rate. The heart has to pump it through the network of blood vessels. In walking, the legs are in motion all the time. Legs have the biggest muscles in the body and walking demands a great deal of blood delivery to the working muscles. In addition, as we walk, the hands swing freely. The hands also have a large number of muscles and these too need blood supply. Hence, the heart has to work hard to supply this blood. Therefore, as we walk, the heart has to beat fast. By working hard, the heart becomes stronger and that is the hallmark of fitness.

Walking

Walking is a simple, healthy and enjoyable activity. When our children take their first steps, we are filled with pleasure and wonderment. Humans have evolved through the ages and gained the ability to walk upright and on two legs. As humans adopted a vertical posture, they were able to see ahead better and had the full freedom to use their hands, making us more creative.

Walking involves using the two legs alternately, with one leg able to support most of the bodyweight at a given time. Walking is different from running as one leg is always touching the ground. In running, there is a phase when both the legs are in the air. We have seen how race walkers walk fast, even faster than many runners, by exaggerating their hip movement to ensure that one leg stays on the ground.

Walking is also a form of exercise that helps us become healthy. Quadriceps are the large muscles at the front of the thighs and hamstrings are the muscles at the back of the thighs. The front muscles help us to straighten the legs and the rear muscles flex the legs. An hour of walking can be a standard measure for calculating how much effort we are putting in. Normally, we can comfortably walk at a speed of 4.5 to 5 kilometres an hour.

As is the case with running, walk wearing shoes that have good cushioning and are comfortable. Though many famous athletes run barefoot and have even won Olympic gold medals (like Abebe Bikila, an Ethiopian who won the Rome Olympic marathon in 1960), I would advise that you wear comfortable shoes when walking. For trekking and hiking, you will need good boots. Choose good footwear for these activities.

Gait While Walking

Each person has a unique gait. In fact, in criminology, detectives are trained to identify a person by his or her walk. There is no need to pay attention to how you walk, so long as you are comfortable. Swing your arms freely as you walk and breathe normally. To check if you are comfortable while walking, start a conversation with your companion. Unlike running, there is no need to warm up before starting a walk. The comfortable feeling of being in the open air without any stress on the body is a unique feature of walking. When you run, you are often required to breathe hard, put in extra effort to maintain a particular speed or to adhere to some rhythmic breathing pattern. No such problems arise when you walk.

Walking as a Route to Fitness

All of us walk every day. To that extent, we all do some exercise. Every housewife does a good deal of walking; maybe she even covers more distance in a day than many people who go out to work. Elderly people who do not step out regularly and are confined to the house for most of the time also do some form of walking. People walk to work or the bus stop or the railway station. In this sense, everyone can claim that he or she is doing a health-building activity. And they are right too. Walking does contribute to fitness. But in this book, we are pursuing a route to aerobic fitness, which is formal, assured and measurable. In this chapter, we will discuss the role of walking as a means of becoming fit.

It is important to have a planned walking programme. This is achievable if you follow the guidelines given in this chapter. But just as a short run to catch a bus is not running for fitness, a casual walk to the market or to drop in on a friend does not count as walking for fitness. Of course, it is possible to integrate your work-related walking into an exercise-oriented programme. For example, if you have to walk more than half an hour regularly to reach your workplace or college or a transit point, you can certainly weave it into your walking routine and take credit for that portion of your walk.

City or Countryside Walking, Trail and Terrain Walking

For convenience, I have divided planned walking into four sections: walking in cities or towns, walking in the countryside, trail walking and terrain walking. Some of these could be interchangeable.

I had once injured my ankle and was forced to switch to walking. I could not bear the load of landing heavily on the ankle while running and the doctor suggested that I should walk instead till the ankle healed. As the injury was not serious, I could walk without difficulty. I could also climb. (I will come to the topic of climbing in the next section of this chapter.) I was amazed at the different pace and effort levels involved in walking. When running, we tend to be focused on our effort and we cannot enjoy much of what goes on around us. But when we walk, we observe the slow-moving landscape, the cart vendor on the street advertising his wares, children hurrying to school and the hustle and bustle of motorists trying to park vehicles in restricted areas. Walking makes us a part of community life.

Walking in Cities

We need to be aware of the dangers of walking on city streets. As vehicular traffic is an ever-present danger to the walker, always walk facing the traffic. That way, you get precious extra seconds to avert accidents. Don't walk in lonely areas, especially after dark. Walking in a group is safe and also fun. Nowadays, there are well-designed walking areas adjacent to most residential colonies. Combinations of residential and commercial areas are ideal for a walking trail. When I was stationed in Delhi, in the 1970s, one of my favourite routes was one from Dhaula Kuan to Greater Kailash and back. Those days the landscape of Delhi was very different from what it is now in 2022. The streets are margined by flyovers, and the architecture has completely changed the scene, vista and panorama of the Delhi that I was familiar with. I sometimes can't find my way around anymore. In those days, you could walk on the roads along with the traffic. While returning from my long walk to Greater Kailash, it used to be a joy to stop for a few minutes at Dhaula Kuan and enjoy a refreshing glass of sugarcane juice. It is also possible to find a big park or recreational area where there are trees, shrubs, bushes and other plant life.

While planning a route to walk on, we must remember that we are working towards a certain objective. We are trying to become fit. This needs a planned approach. Set apart a minimum of 1.5 hours for your daily walk. Anything between 1.5 and 2 hours will count as a walking session.

Walking in the Countryside

In the countryside, it is easy to find woodland that has plenty of trees. A walk of about an hour and a half in such surroundings has double benefits. You, of course, get a vigorous workout. In addition, the oxygen-rich open air, caressed by the trees, is especially beneficial for the lungs.

From 1967 to 1970, I was stationed in Moscow as assistant air force attaché in the Embassy of India. I had fallen ill with a respiratory tract infection and was referred to a Dr Yamschikova. She was the senior lung specialist in a designated government hospital in Moscow. After examining me, she said, 'Mr Iyer, this is a minor infection and you should be all right in a few days. But to regain your strength, you need to go out into the woods and walk every day. Once you have recovered from your present illness, start walking, starting with thirty minutes and bring it up to one and a half hours.' Those days, I was not into any fitness training. However, I followed her advice. Moscow is full of large wooded areas, easily accessible to the motorist. I would walk continuously for about 1.5 hours. I got back to excellent health after four weeks. I mention this incident to stress the importance of walking in wooded areas.

Trail Walking

Trail walking is about locating a site devoted to walkers and joggers. If you live in an area where there are no designated trails, you have to make do with whatever is available in your neighbourhood or within a reasonable motoring distance. The idea is to be away from city traffic and other pollution. In the countryside, it is easy to find such trails. It is invigorating, taking you to clusters of trees and shrubs and maybe even streams and rivulets, making it a pleasurable and satisfying outing. In trail walking, you can concentrate on increasing your walking speed, increasing the length of your stride and setting up a comfortable breathing rhythm – and it will leave you with a feeling of having carried out robust conditioning. An hour and a half of trail walking gives you an excellent workout. Let me tell you about my memorable trail walking experience. In January 2011, I was in Washington DC for a few months. The Great Falls area near DC has a very well-designed trail stretching over 20 kilometres. It has up and down gradients and offers great scenic views. My granddaughter Tara, grandson Venkat and their mother, Indira, decided to tackle the trail on an invigorating January morning. I was eighty-one years old then but went through the full circuit offered by the trail. The children took off at a fast clip but I gamely kept up, resting often and enjoying the vista and the landscape, which also included a rivulet. Indira, very fit, proceeded at my pace, keeping an eye on me. The trail took about 5 hours to complete, and we caught up with the children well before the end. Both are top athletes and must have done a few extra kilometres, going ahead and retracing their steps along some routes.

Terrain Walking

Terrain, in the context of walking, is an area with different gradients, giving us a variety of surfaces and at diverse angles – little climbs interspersed with downward pathways. This kind of walk gives an excellent training effect to the heart, keeping the heart rate fairly high for a continuous period. The different muscles in the legs are also made to work, which makes them rugged. If you like an additional load on your body (the more the load, the more the benefit, up to a point at least), you can wear a weighted belt, like I used to do during my runs. Good sports shops stock up on devices like weighted armlets, to make it more challenging and therefore enhancing the benefits of the workout. An upward gradient will increase the benefits of the walk. If you live in a city, you can simulate terrain walking by choosing flyovers. In Delhi, the Safdarjung Flyover was my favourite spot. I would go up the flyover, walk down comfortably and retrace my steps. An hour and a half of this up and down walk is demanding and beneficial.

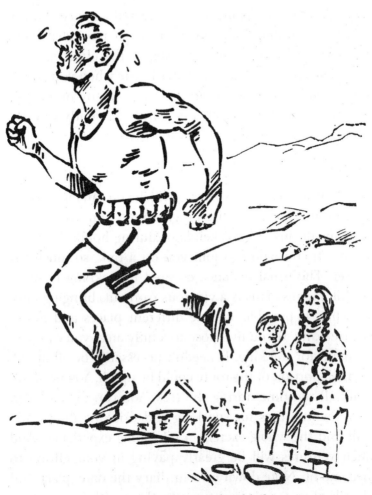

Running with a weighted belt.

Mix up all the types of walks mentioned above. It will add variety and take the boredom away from your exercise sessions. Keep a journal and write a brief account of the extent of your workout: the duration, route and any observations about the workout. Try not to pause while walking. Maintain a constant speed. Note down your pulse at the end of each exercise session. Remember that you are on a planned and targeted activity and not a casual saunter. Your diary will be a reminder about the number of workouts, the speed, the effort and the experience. Always carry a water bottle when you go out on a walking session. Strap it on or use any number of devices available to carry water. Drink frequently, whether you feel thirsty or not. Hydration is vital.

Trekking

Trekking is a planned workout, which you can incorporate into your regular exercise programme as an extra effort, perhaps during the weekends or during holidays. If you have a friend who can join you on a trek, so much the better. The usual distance covered in trekking is about 25 kilometres. This is a vigorous workout, bringing huge benefits. If possible, choose different places and routes for trekking. If you live close to a hilly area, you can plan a circuit for trekking. It needn't necessarily be all uphill. A small portion of the route could be uphill. You need not walk all the time during the trek. You can take a break of a few minutes for snacking and drinking fluids. You will find the whole exercise a refreshing experience. And such ventures will be greatly paying in your efforts to become fit. Note down in your diary the date, place and details of your trek, and compare them with future treks. You should be doing a trek at least once in two months. Trekking, however, should not be considered part of your daily walking commitment; it should be regarded as a bonus.

Speed and Load While Walking

You should try to increase the speed of your walking, at least two or three times a week. After all, we are trying to become fitter, and we need to step up the load on the body. Another method of raising the load on the body is power walking, where you carry a light load in your hands while walking. It could be a pair of light dumbbells (1 kg each will do). Or you can buy a pair of armlets, which you can strap on to your wrists with a small weight attached. Don't try to use heavy weights, especially in the initial stages of your walking workouts. One kg in each hand is ample for taking on a load in power walking. You will be surprised to see your heart rate going up. You will also feel the extra effort on your body. In your first few weeks of power walking, keep the exercise to 20 or 25 minutes. As you get familiar with the load, you can gradually increase it to 45 minutes. Do not practise this form of walking for longer than that. And indulge in power walking not more than twice a week.

I can confirm from my experience that walking in any form is as good as running for becoming and remaining fit. A small injury (when I was fifty-six years old) had forced me to switch over from running to walking. I had walked for about three months, mostly doing trail walking, in Nagpur and a few weeks in Delhi. In Nagpur, I used to live in a hilly area called Seminary Hills. There were plenty of routes to choose from, consisting of up and down gradients. I used to walk 10 to 12 kilometres a day, starting from the Air Force Station, going down to the Gondwana Club and back. Occasionally, I would take the highway to Amaravati, do a 4-miler and come back, a total of 8 miles. From my journal, I can see the types of workouts I did at any time in the past. I can also see that I had maintained the same level of fitness as when I was running, by comparing the various parameters that indicate robust health. These include low pulse, maintenance of low weight, general health, appetite, etc. (Yes, I do note down all details in my journal.)

Climbing

Climbing can be an alternative route to fitness. It is a vigorous activity. Any movement against gravity is strenuous. In fact, in physics, only if you have moved something up or down can it be defined as work. Any movement along a horizontal plane is not considered work. But this definition has no significance in physical training, as we all know that we do very strenuous work along a horizontal plane when we run, walk, etc.

In climbing, your legs become strong. As you may have noticed, people living in hilly regions have very strong and robust lower legs. Their hearts too would be automatically strong. The only problem in adopting climbing as a regular exercise plan is the need for a suitable terrain. You need to be in hilly terrain. An occasional planned vacation may allow you to climb, and it is well worth trying.

Climbing Ropes

Incidentally, climbing ropes is an effective exercise for the upper body. One can tie a coir rope on a branch of a tree. Param and I would often climb and reach the top, maybe at a height of 4 metres. It is a demanding exercise and requires great upper body strength. If you can climb a rope, you can do several pull-ups too. Initially, you have to keep on trying till you can go up 1 metre. It is all about practice and you will gradually be able to do more.

Swimming

Swimming is an excellent exercise. When you swim, all your limbs work vigorously. The special advantage of swimming is that the limbs are predominantly underwater and work with buoyancy, under reduced gravitational pull. This reduces the effort required to move the limbs, giving you a workout that does not demand too much effort. In fact, physiotherapists often advise patients to move an injured limb underwater, without the trauma of weight-bearing.

I am a good swimmer. While learning to swim, in a big temple tank in Kozhikode, Kerala, I would carry a couple of dried coconut shells strung together with a coir rope. That was my lifeguard; it kept me floating, freeing both hands to strike out and attempt to swim. When I had learned the rudiments of swimming and could swim without the help of my lifeguard, I would attempt to swim as far into the water as possible. Within a month of learning to swim, I could swim right across the width of the tank, which was a good 100 metres long. I have also swum in the sea in Kozhikode and enjoyed it. The beach there is quiet without any great tidal disturbance, and devoid of sharks. I have also swum in rivers, in the Palghat River when young and in the Yamuna when I was in service and was commanding an Air Force unit in Manauri, a village near Allahabad (now Prayagraj).

The main advantage of swimming over other forms of exercise is the therapeutic effect it gives, leaving your muscles relaxed at the end of the workout. As far as possible, every parent should try to get their child to learn how to swim. I was lucky to get a national swimming coach to train my two daughters. I taught my son to swim when he was five years old. All three learned to swim within two to three weeks. Decades later I had the special pleasure of teaching my grandchildren to swim. Now it is the turn of my great-grandchildren to swim. I am eager to take up the training myself, but perhaps not unreasonably, their parents are reluctant to get them trained by a ninety-two-year-old!

Swimming as an exercise to achieve fitness is carried out like any other form of exercise. An hour of swimming, at various speeds and with different techniques, is ideal. Allot 10 to 15 minutes for crawl, breaststroke, butterfly and backstroke. Try a few jumps and dives. If you want to become an expert swimmer, take instructions from a competent coach. Swimming should be carried out, like any other form of exercise, regularly, at least five times a week.

It is always a good idea to learn life-saving techniques from an expert; you never know when they will come in useful. Someone saved me in the Kozhikode tank when I had just learned the basics of swimming, at the age of seven. I was tired, and away from the steps of the tank. After joining the Air Force, I learned life-saving skills at an event organized by St. John Ambulance in Chennai. It was a one-week course, and we were thoroughly drilled into various methods of saving people from drowning. One technique that particularly struck me is the McGreggor grip, which is used when the victim is likely to hold on tightly to you, the rescuer, and hamper your rescue effort and put you in danger too! In my turn, I have saved an adult swimmer when he was tiring in the Manauri swimming pool. Talking about life-saving, I must mention here an unforgettable and consequential moment in Delhi when my son was five years old. I had taught him to swim in the Air Force swimming pool. After a week of training, Param was getting the hang of swimming, and he wanted to show off his skills to his sisters. My daughters had already learned to swim, and the family drove down to the Air Force pool. By the time I had parked the car and was approaching the pool, the children were at the pool, and Param had jumped in, but at the deep end. As with all accidents, everything happened in a flash. My son was struggling at the unexpected downward draft after his jump and unable to muster his recently learned floating and stroking skills. He was clearly in distress and Mina, all of ten years, jumped right in after him and pulled him to the side easily. All this, just as I was approaching them after parking the car. As I was saying, life-saving skills are very useful.

As with other forms of exercise, maintain a journal and record your speed, type of swimming, etc., every time you work out. It will be an invaluable reference and anecdotal record. We need to practise personal hygiene whenever we swim, like showering before and after a swim and using clean towels. One must also look out for the bleaching powder solution that is released into swimming pools to clean them. My grandson Shankar had a habit of opening his eyes underwater, presumably, as he once explained to me, to observe underwater animal life. One day, when we were leaving the pool after an hour of training, Shankar complained that his eyes were hurting badly. His eyes were bloodshot. I realized he had been underwater near a tube that was delivering a bleach powder solution to the pool, and he must have received a big dose of bleaching powder in his eyes. It took my doctor friend Mohan Kumar a good half hour to wash his eyes and remove the corrosive agent.

Cycling

Cycling stands apart as a vigorous, interesting, convenient and pleasurable form of fitness-building activity. I have done my share of cycling and can say from experience that it gives a great workout, without too heavy a load on the legs. As the body weight is borne by the gluteus muscles at the waist, the legs are free to exert their maximum, without the task of weight-bearing. Race biking is a great sport and the Tour de France is one of the greatest sporting events, which demands extraordinary stamina and fitness. But here we are discussing cycling as a fitness-building exercise, and your choice of a bicycle depends on whether you want to indulge in track cycling or road. There are special bikes for use on the track. But a regular cycle perhaps with a few gears is generally the best buy for most of us. The gears will be useful when doing long road work.

When I was a wing commander and posted in Delhi, I used to cycle to work. But these were short 30-minute rides and could not be counted as part of my fitness regime. When I was serving in Nagpur a few years later, I used to cycle for 1.5 hours, which qualifies as a fitness exercise. Amravati Road was my favourite cycling route. As I was going through a period of knee rehabilitation, the doctor recommended cycling in place of my regular running. I would load the saddle with my 5 kg belt for additional load and set up a good pace. The cyclist always needs to be cautious about traffic when riding on roads. The only way to avoid traffic is to cycle on a dedicated cycle track. But that luxury is perhaps available only in big cities or in the countryside. Of course, all cyclists must wear a helmet when out on the roads.

The advantage of cycling over running is that we can avoid weight bearing on the legs. Cycling is a concentrated form of toughening the upper and lower leg muscles and loading the heart. If you are facing an upwards gradient, you can always change gear and cruise. Or if the mood takes you, you can pedal harder and climb up the gradient for a strenuous workout.

The advice given when starting running, regarding warm-ups, applies to cycling too. But you can warm up on the bike itself if you start pedalling slowly and work up your speed gradually. Cooling down can be done by reducing the speed for the last 5 minutes. If you cycle to work regularly, you can credit it towards your fitness efforts, provided an average trip is at least 40 minutes long. Short trips of 20 minutes would not count as fitness building.

A stationary bike is a useful piece of equipment to have. You can then, in the comfort of your home, work on it at your convenience. You can adjust the speed, set the degree of difficulty and, of course, you are safe from the hazards of the road. As always, keep a record of your workouts in your journal, including details of time, distance and heart rate at the end of the session.

Aerobic Dancing

I must confess that I have never tried aerobic dancing and my knowledge and understanding are limited to my reading and observation. Some of the gyms that I have frequented offered aerobic dancing sessions. I could see that all participants had an excellent and even demanding load on their limbs and heart. I do not doubt that they got great aerobic benefits from it. It is also a pleasurable and socially satisfying form of group exercise.

Treadmill

I have been working out in gyms for more than three decades. The treadmill is an excellent method of obtaining a robust workout at your convenience. You can work at it in a controlled fashion. You can choose your speed and control the degree of difficulty by increasing or decreasing the gradient. The treadmill also records your pulse rate. While exercising on a treadmill, you can watch a video of your choice or even get important work done. For all these reasons, the treadmill is a versatile station in your quest for fitness. An added advantage is that it gives you the option of choosing a convenient time for your daily exercise, and this is important for all working people.

Conclusion

In this chapter, I discussed alternative methods of gaining fitness. The reader would have noticed that in every method the crucial element is a movement of the limbs, continuously for some time, usually an hour or more. The aim is always to make the heart work harder and harder. The heart will then serve you efficiently, and you will be active enough to cope with any form of emergency. The human body is designed in such a way that with an activity, the muscles (including the heart, which is a muscle) grow strong, and in the absence of any activity, they rust. If an idle mind is the devil's workshop, an idle body is the devil's den. The mantra to keep in mind when seeking fitness is to be on the MOVE.

FIVE

Strength, Flexibility and Injury Prevention

In this chapter, we shall discuss two aspects of fitness: strength and flexibility. We shall also see the importance of avoiding injuries.

Midlife Crisis

I would like to start by touching upon midlife crisis when we start worrying about the state of our health and fitness. Midlife crisis usually affects people between the ages of 45 and 65 when they are at the peak of their career. Childhood and youth have passed by and we start wondering about our mortality, state of health, unfinished work and responsibility. We are also concerned about our work, profession, family and social relationships, etc. In this section, I will deal with the fitness aspect of this condition.

We are often flooded with information about regaining fitness and strength. Print and television media frequently discuss fitness-related topics. Social media too remains active on this topic as it is of interest to most of us. How do we process this abundance of information?

The universal consensus of all the research and studies is that exercise has a beneficial effect on fitness and longevity, and helps to ward off the ill effects of ageing. There is of course conflicting advice on the type, intensity and duration of exercise. There are also warnings about overdoing exercises. While all this is interesting information to us, it does sometimes leave us confused. The mere volume and content of data are daunting, and often contradictory.

Antonin Scalia, the American Supreme Court Judge, said in one of his judgements, 'If there is no correct answer to a question, then any particular answer cannot be termed wrong.' In the context of exercise, this statement can be rephrased as: if there is no laid-down rule as to the correct amount and type of exercise for a person, then any opinion on the subject cannot be termed wrong. Our common sense tells us that exercise is beneficial and keeps at bay problems associated with ageing. This is where I think I can give some guidance. I have been in this business of seeking information on fitness, and have been a practitioner of the art of becoming and remaining fit for several decades.

I have found that exercise is a panacea for many age-related problems. When you go outdoors for a walk, you come back refreshed, and any lingering tiredness or even headache disappears. And if you make walking a regular habit, you proactively prevent any malaise from cropping up. The same is true if you take part in any other form of exercise. The magic of exercise has convinced me that age is just a number, and we could be as fit as required, at any age. I have been encouraged to hold this opinion by my daughter Indira Jayaraman.

My daughter Indu, a fitness enthusiast in her own right, has come up with a theory about ageing. She says that the cells in our body are basically like obedient sheep. They just do the job that they are assigned. For example, the muscles in our legs consist of millions of cells. The job of these cells is to contract, in a coordinated way, so that the legs can move. All they know, and all they need to know, is how to do their job. To do their job well, they need to have the fuel (glycogen) and oxygen to burn that fuel. These two items are supplied to them by the heart through the blood vessels. When you are in your seventies, say, the cells will continue to contract, as they are designed to do, provided they get the blood supply. In this theory, the conclusion is that you can continue to employ your legs efficiently, at any age, if your heart functions well. The cells in the legs do not know how old you are; whether you are a young person or in your eighties. To some extent, I agree with this theory because I am an example of its veracity. I can bend or extend my leg easily at the age of ninety-two. My leg muscles are very strong. I have made it my business to keep them strong all through the past decades by working regularly on them and by using my legs every day for running.

At the same time, I am also the victim of a progressive illness called osteoarthritis. In this disease, the soft lining between bones wears away, making the bones (here, the bones in the upper and lower legs) rub against each other, producing pain. So, in me, you see an example of strong legs (helping to move with efficiency) coexisting with arthritis (which makes movement painful). I have, therefore, modified my view. Ageing is a fact of life. It affects all living things. It is true that by proper exercise, we can ward off many of the manifestations of ageing, but we cannot completely escape from the ravages of ageing.

So while an older person's cells are less robust and have less energy than a younger person's cells, we can delay their degeneration by exercise. So all is not lost. I would like to conclude this section on an optimistic note. It is my firm belief, based on my long experience in experimenting with activities that promote fitness and also on the bulk of scientific research on the benefits of exercise, that all of us can keep at bay the ill effects of ageing by exercising. It is possible to enjoy the comparatively leisurely pace of senior citizenship, reduce the chances of falling ill and prolong our lifespan.

But the questions remain. How much exercise? What intensity? How often? What happens when you are not well? Which exercise? Let me answer these questions, so that you can draw up a plan to start your fitness regime. Incidentally, I have already answered the last question, regarding which exercise. Any of the exercises mentioned in chapters 3 and 4, or a combination of exercises, is good for you. They all lead you to aerobic fitness.

How Much Exercise?

Regarding how much you need to exercise, I have indicated, at each stage, how much is needed to remain fit. But, being normal human beings, we may not be able to sustain exercise for 1.5 hours on every occasion. So here is a practical suggestion. Keep 1.5 hours as a target. If you are unable to work up to that time, so be it. Do what you can, log it in your journal and come back to it another day. Do not try to make up the lost time by exercising extra. That will be counterproductive. And it may lead to fatigue. There is no point in worrying about falling behind on your schedule. Life is full of uncertainties, and the events of a day may take you away from your fitness regime. Your fitness is not going to suffer from an occasional lapse. I was once a victim of not following this advice. I was travelling from Chennai to Delhi by train and I missed a day of running. The next day, I tried to run an extra 2 hours, to make up for the lost day, and got so fatigued that I had to rest for a full week to recover. If you miss a day, so be it. Try to be as regular as possible. As a general principle, if you are running, a minimum of 20 minutes will count for exercise benefits. If you are walking, a minimum of 40 minutes will count as exercise.

Intensity

Speed is not important when you are running. Comfort is. In Chapter 3, I have discussed the talk test. You should be able to carry on a conversation, without getting out of breath when you are running. You are not in a race; you are not competing against anyone. So enjoy your jogs. The same principle applies when you are cycling, swimming or climbing. You should get the feeling of working out in comfort. You should cut back if you feel the load of the exercise.

How Often?

In the pursuit of exercise, how often is an important question. Exercise should be regular, not sporadic. It is always better to do moderate exercise regularly rather than do a Herculean effort, followed by long gaps. Five days a week is what we should aim for. I run seven days a week and gym six days a week. You may say I can maintain this schedule because I am old and have nothing much else to do. But let me assure you I keep busy with many activities, including writing this book on fitness. So it is up to you to decide how often you plan to work out a week. But it should not be less than three days a week to get optimum benefits.

What Happens When You Are Not Well?

All of us fall ill some time or other. Yes, I too have fallen ill, but rarely. When that happens, it is prudent to take a rest till you recover, and continue to rest for a few days after recovery. Discretion and prudence should govern our activities. Even a cold or mild fever should not be ignored. The body is giving us a warning that all is not well, and we should heed this warning. A rough and ready method of returning to an exercise regime is that we should take rest, after recovery, for the same number of days that we had been sick. Your journal can often guide you as to what kind and intensity of exercise you had been following before you fell sick. It might give clues of overexertion. This is one of the many advantages of maintaining a journal.

Now that we have had a review of how to plan our fitness-building activities, let us continue with some other aspects of fitness, which need our attention.

Strength

Strength is a term applied to our muscles. The human body consists of three types of muscles: the voluntary muscles, smooth muscles and cardiac muscles. Smooth muscles perform involuntary functions like pushing food through our intestines, increasing the size of the pupils of the eyes in the dark, etc. We have no control over these muscles. But what we can control is the voluntary muscles. Our limbs are endowed with voluntary muscles. We can move these muscles, as per our requirement. In this section on strength, we are concerned with voluntary muscles. These are muscles of our legs, arms, shoulders, etc. These muscles help us to move or perform various actions such as walking, running, cycling, climbing, pulling, pushing and lifting. Our ability to carry out everyday tasks depends upon the strength of the voluntary muscles. To be fit, we need to keep these muscles as strong as possible.

The strength of our muscles starts to decrease, as we age. It is estimated that our strength starts reducing at the rate of 10 per cent every decade, starting from the age of thirty. In other words, if we do not make an effort to retain our strength, we would have lost half of our strength by the time we are eighty years old. But with strength-building exercises, we can retard the progressive loss of strength. For example, even at the age of eighty or ninety, we can retain as much strength as a sixty-year-old.

We have seen that aerobic fitness is the most important form of fitness because our very existence depends on the heart, lungs and blood vessels functioning properly. But to be aerobically fit, you need to move your legs and arms. And that needs strength. Strength can be defined as the capacity of our limbs to perform, without strain, tasks assigned to our muscles in our daily life. Walking, running, climbing, swimming and carrying heavy objects, all these tasks require strong limbs. The science of human biology tells us that our muscles become strong by working against a progressive load. As we use our muscles to carry bigger and bigger loads, the muscle fibres break down and rebuild themselves more strongly. This is the method of making our muscles stronger.

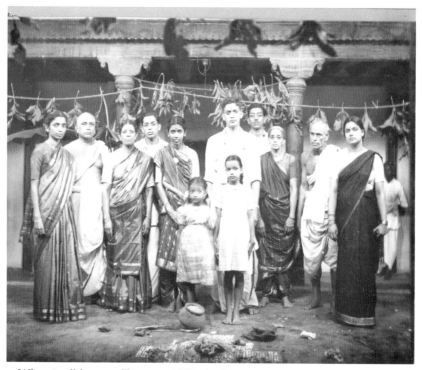

When it all began – Tirupati, 1953. Author P.V. Iyer and his bride, Kalyani.
(*Left to right*) Kalyani's sister, parents, two brothers, author's parents and sister.

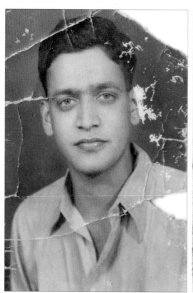

The picture that the author's wife,
Kalyani (Kay), kept in her handbag
for 57 years.

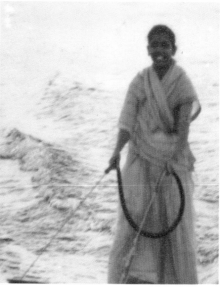

Adventurous Kay – Water-surfing in the
Dal Lake, Srinagar, 1959.

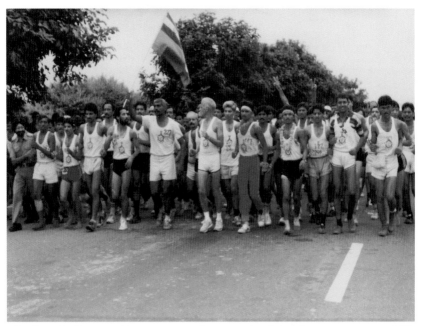

The Agra–Delhi run – 300 runners took part in this 240-kilometre event in 1985.

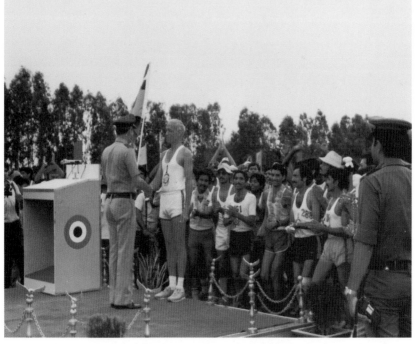

The author, Air Marshal P.V. Iyer, at the end of the Agra–Delhi run, handing over the Air Force flag to the Air Chief, Air Marshal Denis La Fontaine, on Air Force Day, 8 October 1985.

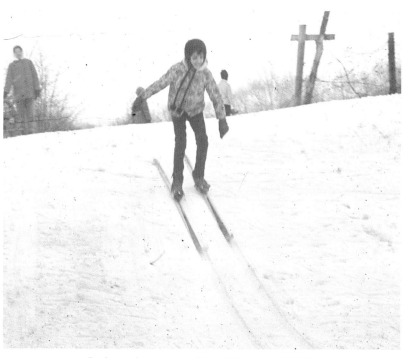

Indu – the expert skier, Moscow, 1968.

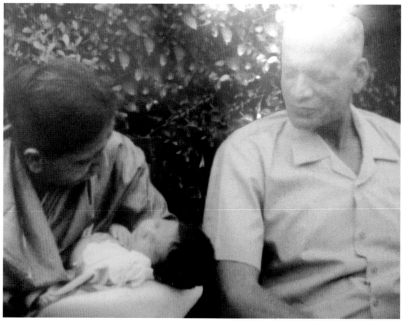

The joys of grandparenting – Kay and the author with their
eldest grandchild, Shankar.

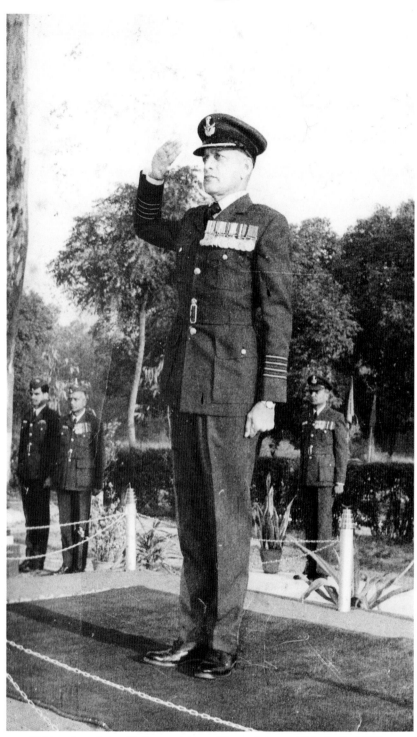

Taking the salute, Air Force station, Manauri (near Allahabad), 1978.

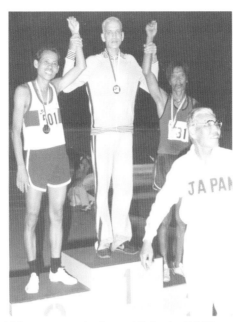

Fifty-one-year-old Iyer – catapulted to gold! At the 5,000-metre running race: Singapore Asian Veterans' Athletic Meet, September 1981.

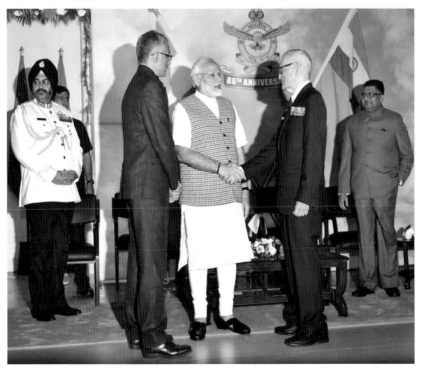

The author with Prime Minister Narendra Modi and Air Chief Marshal B.S. Dhanoa – on Air Force Day, 8 October 2018, at Air House, Delhi.

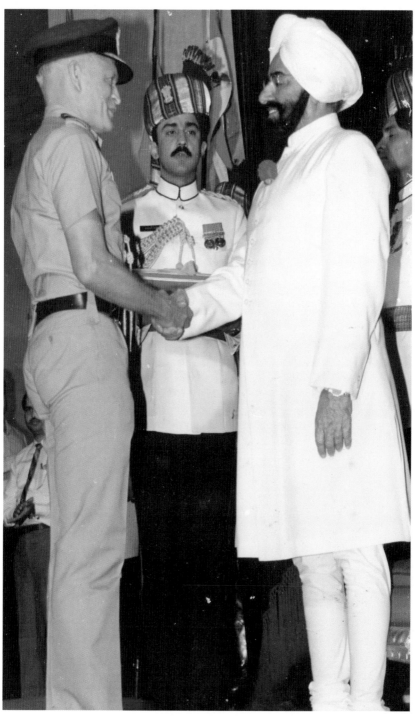

Air Marshal P.V. Iyer receiving the Ati Vishisht Seva Medal (AVSM) from the President of India, 1986.

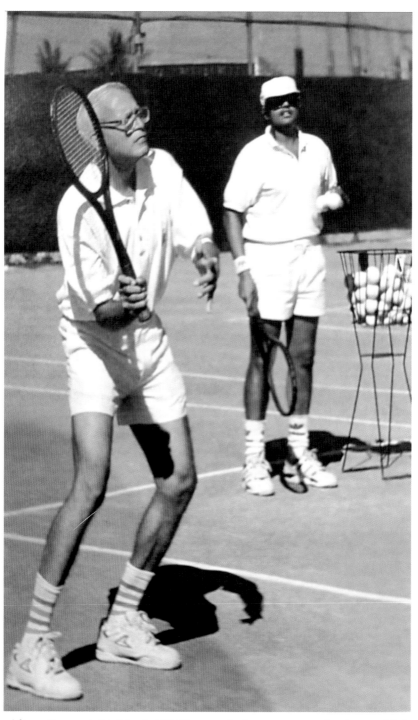

After retirement, Air Marshal P.V. Iyer coached youngsters under the watchful eye of Ramesh Krishnan, at the Krishnan Tennis Centre, Chennai, 1996.

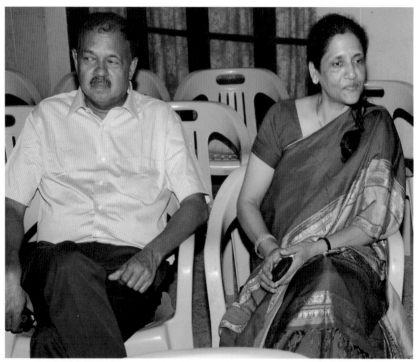

Mina, the author's eldest, with her husband, Anand.

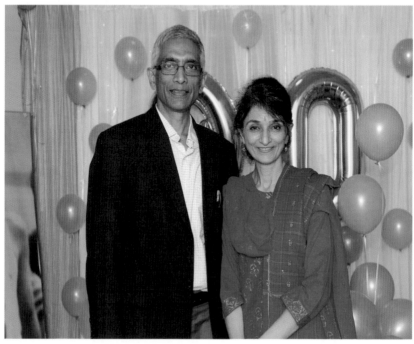

Parameswaran Iyer, a civil servant, the author's youngest, with wife, Indira.

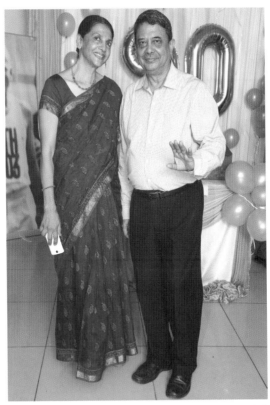

Indira, the author's second daughter, with her husband, Lt Col. Jayaraman.

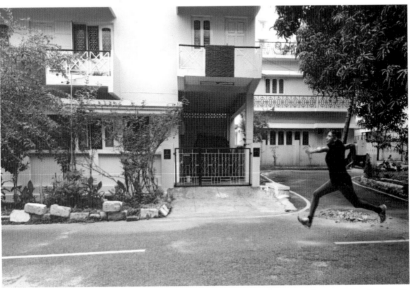

Indira Jayaraman, at sixty-three years, during a moment in the sprint phase of her daily run (2020). *Note:* The leg split and the stride length convey speed.

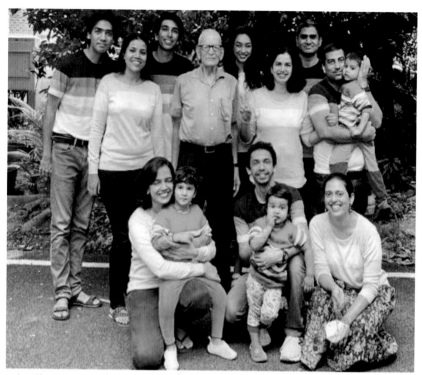

An illustrious patriarch – the author (*centre*) with his grandchildren and their spouses around him. (*Left to right, standing*) Ashwin, Kamini, Venkat, Tara, Janaki, Ashwin, Ashwath. (*Left to right, sitting*) Akila, Shankar, Sneha. The photo also includes the author's three great-grandchildren (*left to right*) Vara, Anika and Aarav.

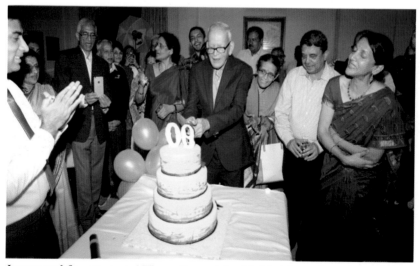

Joyous and fit – at ninety! The author cutting his birthday cake, surrounded by his cheering family. Defence Club, RSI, Bangalore, 2019.

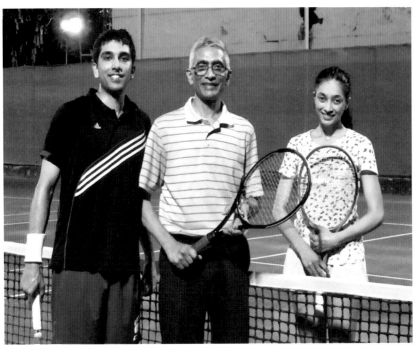

Param Iyer – The Road Manager – for his two professional tennis-playing children, Tara and Venkat.

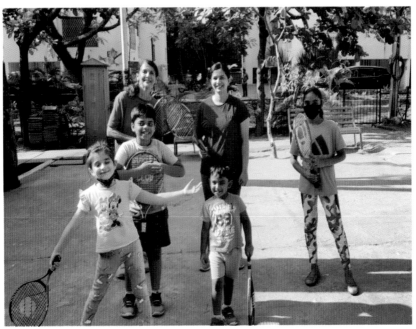

Courtside – Indira's tennis school, Sena Vihar, Bangalore, 2022.
Indira, with assistant coach, daughter, Janaki.

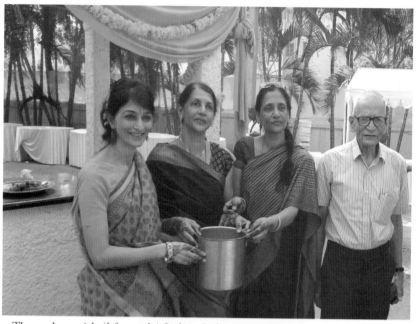

The author, with (*left to right*) Indira, Indu and Mina, at his granddaughter's wedding, Bangalore, 2015.

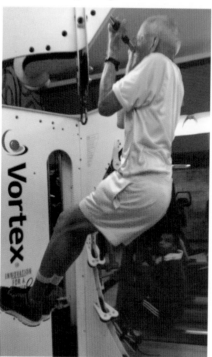

Uplift your life – the author, enjoying pull-ups at age ninety.

Importance of Strength Training

Muscular strength is an important tool to maintain vigorous fitness. Strong muscles help us to perform various activities without strain. They help us by preventing injuries and protecting vital organs from getting damaged while we perform our daily activities. Strong muscles keep our metabolic rate high, preventing obesity. Latest theories assert that efforts to strengthen our muscles directly contribute to warding off cancer, diabetes and cardiovascular diseases. They also increase our lifespan. I am a firm believer in this theory. It is my conviction that working out in a gym for the last four or five decades has helped me maintain my strength and warded off potential diseases. Along with my running training every day, strength training has made me fit. I can use 7.5 kg dumbbells in my workouts regularly and bench press 30 kg. Due to the COVID-19 pandemic, I have not visited a gym in two years, but I have set up a home gym, with all the minimum requirements, where I work out six days a week. I shall explain how to set up such a home gym without too much effort or expense.

Training for Strength

In my experiments with strength training, I have realized that progressive resistance training exercise is the way to go to become strong. This can take many forms and some of the popular methods of gaining strength include lifting weights, working on various gym machines, using a flexible band and isometric exercises. Visit a regular gym if you can and work out there at least four times a week. You can also take advantage of the trained coaches present in gyms. You can use the available machines and weights to strengthen all the muscle groups of your body, and the coach can guide you on the types of exercises you should do, the number of repetitions, the number of sets, etc. But make sure that the coach does not hurry you to make progress. Coaches often tend to encourage their trainees to progress fast, partly to show off their prowess as a coach. Go at your own pace. Your aim is not to become strong overnight but to develop an exercise regime for life. Always remember that your workouts are a process, a journey and not a destination.

Home Gym

For some of us, it is difficult to go to a gym regularly, more so in these times of the pandemic, a complex and unpredictable affliction. If you cannot or do not want to visit a gym, you can easily set up a home gym. I have set up one that is adequate for all my needs of strength training. All you need to buy are a few inexpensive pieces of equipment. Let me list them for you:

1. A set of dumbbells, ranging from 2 kg to 10 kg
2. Two sets of ankle straps weighing between 2 kg and 5 kg
3. A set of terra bands of varying degrees of resistance

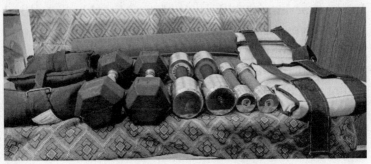

Home gym – minimum equipment

4. A floor mat
5. A small, narrow workout bench (5 feet × 15 inches)
6. A small stool, about 15 inches high

Exercises

I suggest that you do a set of exercises that are required to engage all the major muscle groups in your body. Remember you are not training to take part in a bodybuilding competition. You are trying to become fit and remain fit. For that purpose, a few simple exercises, carried out regularly four or five times a week are ample. The only point to remember is that you should be regular in your workouts. You cannot store strength, just as you cannot store fitness. You have to earn it every week. One or two weeks of rest is OK. But you should soon get back to your training routine. The best method of learning is from an experienced person who has worked out in a gym. However, see Appendix for a list of some exercises you can do.

Flexibility Exercises

Flexibility is an important component of fitness. It helps us make full use of our muscles, leading to an economy of effort. It also helps prevent injury. It is easy to perform exercises related to flexibility because they do not involve any weights. Some of them are performed standing, while others are done sitting and some lying down. But these are as important as strengthening exercises. Flexibility improves the way we do work and prevents injuries. They should cover all the major joints of the body. See Appendix for a list of flexibility exercises that you can do.

Preventing Injury

Strong muscles and regular stretching exercises prevent
injuries. Never start any exercise programme, whether
running or cycling or swimming, without a proper warm-
up. The same goes for weight training. Ease into the
exercise gradually. Use smaller weights in the beginning
and move up to heavier weights gradually.

I am guilty of ignoring this on a few occasions. When I
was living in Delhi, I used to take part in a weekly running
race, known as the Otto Peltzer Race. It was in honour
of a German athletic coach, who trained athletes free at
the National Stadium, at the eastern end of Rajpath. It
was conducted every Sunday at 7 a.m. It was an informal
race, with no officials, and about thirty athletes would
turn up, including some soldiers from the Raj Rif Centre
in Delhi Cantonment. Ranjit Bhatia, an Olympic athlete
and professor of mathematics at St. Stephen's College,
was another regular. We would warm up and someone
would say, 'Get set and go.' All of us would run as fast
as we could to Rajpath, around India Gate, and onwards
to Rashtrapati Bhavan. We would climb up the Raisina
Hills, touch the grilled gates of the President's Residence
and run back to the National Stadium and the starting
point. It was a 7-kilometre-long race. It is a demanding
race, especially the steep climb near Rashtrapati Bhavan.
I would normally complete the race in 27 minutes, at a
pace of under 4 minutes a kilometre. Ranjit Bhatia would
be ahead by a good 100 metres. The young athletes would
do it much faster, and we all enjoyed the camaraderie and
tea afterwards.

On one such occasion, I was able to cut down my
race time by a good 15 seconds. A sports reporter was

covering the event and he, on learning that I was sixty years old and could do the 7 kilometres in less than 27 minutes, wished to take a video of my running. I happily agreed and sprinted for about 50 metres without any warm-up or stretching. And sure enough, I injured my hamstring. Hamstring injuries take several weeks to heal and I had to stop my training and get into rehab mode. An important marathon race was scheduled the next month, and there was no way I could train for it or compete in it. I am narrating this incident to send out a message to all fitness enthusiasts that never attempt any serious exercise programme without a proper warm-up. In my excitement to show off to the media, I had injured myself.

All this is to emphasize that injury prevention is a matter of proper warm-up, gradual increase in load or speed, and proper adherence to stretching and strengthening.

In ending this chapter on strength training, let me remind you that strength training will pay good dividends as we approach middle age and plan to ward off the ravages of time by counterattacking.

SIX

A Sound Mind in a Sound Body

We have talked about physical fitness, but we all know that mental fitness is equally important. The prerequisite for a healthy mind is a healthy body. We have had sufficient discussion about keeping the body healthy. Let us now discuss the mind with the understanding that we are doing our best to keep the body sound.

The principle of engaging the body is equally applicable to the mind too. Employ the mind to keep it healthy. But there is a slight difference between the body and the mind. It is possible to be completely lazy and do nothing with the limbs. But the mind is almost always active, except when we sleep. What we then do with our minds becomes important. Constructive, creative thoughts nourish the mind. All of us, in the course of pursuing our profession or business or other daily tasks, employ our brains on a variety of issues and problems to take appropriate decisions. This is part of our regular work. In addition, we need to challenge our brains with thoughts not related to our profession.

You can, on your own, device any number of schemes, invent new methods of occupying your mind, constantly challenging, constantly asking your mind to innovate, to be creative, to bring in different approaches to problem-solving. The brain benefits from such challenges.

Scientists tell us that challenges to the brain improve the connectivity of the brain and prevent age-related deterioration, like memory loss.

The mind and the body are so closely connected that we consider them together when discussing overall fitness. When both function well, we can lead a happy and productive life. Any impairment in one will have an adverse influence on the other. While problems of the body are evident, those of the mind are generally more complex and not easily detectable. The field of psychiatry deals with diagnosing and treating mental disorders. The only time I had to consult a psychiatrist was when I was serving at Pondicherry University, as the Director of Sports, NSS and students welfare.

One day, there was an anonymous letter on my office table that said because of my alleged losses in the stock market, my composure had been affected and so had my interaction with my colleagues. As with many anonymous letters, it had an element of truth. I had invested in the stock market. But contrary to what the letter said I had made a small profit. However, as I was not used to any criticism regarding my public behaviour, the letter and its content disturbed my mind. I talked about this to a young physician friend, who was doing his postgraduation in psychiatry at the Jawaharlal Nehru Institute of Postgraduate Medical Education and Research. I told him it had made me brood and had adversely affected my generally calm attitude. The young doctor, who often accompanied me on my runs, was genuinely surprised. He told me I was an inspiration to him and other youth who worked out at the university grounds and gym. He said, 'Sir, in fact, if I have any worries, I would come straight to you for guidance and comfort. And here you are, asking my advice!' He suggested that I ignore the anonymous letter and continue mentoring young people. This piece of advice from my young friend wiped out the lingering unease in my mind in a trice, and I was my normal calm self again. As this incident illustrates, small matters sometimes affect our minds, and it is important to consult a friend or a doctor to help us regain our poise.

According to scientists, our brain is more competent than the fastest computer created by humans. It is also said that we use only a very small percentage of the capacity of our brain. Perhaps as little as 5 per cent. When we learn a language or learn to play a musical instrument, or study, we are training our mind; the mind can take in an almost limitless amount of knowledge and skill. A child can learn to speak several languages without difficulty. Even in old age, our brain can assimilate new knowledge and learn new skills.

In this chapter, I shall give examples of our body's ability to support and encourage the various activities that the mind wants to indulge in. I have to fall back on events that have taken place in my close family circle. My intention is not to boast about my family's achievements, and I hope you will be able to relate to these episodes.

I have always been fond of learning new languages. As a young officer in the Air Force, I started learning French. In those days, we had no concept of remote learning or the internet. The best I could do was borrow some old gramophone records that were in French with supporting text. The Air Force didn't expect me to learn French or any other language. It was just my desire to study something out of the ordinary. In the freezing cold of Srinagar, I would wake up early and study French from 4 a.m. to 6 a.m. before going to the Air Force base.

I then found a Dutch priest, Father Byfoet, in the Burn Hall School in Srinagar, who knew French. He agreed to give me tuition in French, three times a week, at the princely sum of ₹20 a month! After work, I would cycle down to the Burn Hall School in the evenings, meet him and spend an hour learning French with the young man. I was eventually able to pass the interpretership examination in French, conducted by the School of Foreign Languages under the Ministry of Defence. I was even employed as an interpreter by the Directorate of Intelligence at the Air Headquarters in Delhi. I earned the nickname 'Frenchy' among my friends in the Air Force. After I had retired from service, I joined the Alliance Francaise in Pondicherry, refreshed my French and earned the 'Diplome de Langue' degree. I also learned some German and passed preliminary exams in that language, while in service. But the progress I made in learning Russian is worth narrating. I had studied Russian on my own, again borrowing some gramophone records. This was one of the reasons that I was posted to Russia as assistant air force attaché in the Embassy of India in Moscow. There, I had diplomatic status, and the protocol demanded that I be presented to the dean of protocol in the Russian Foreign Office. Dressed in ceremonial Air Force uniform with trimmings of gold, my boss, Air Commodore Achreja and I drove down to the Foreign Office and were ushered in to meet General Russikov. The General spoke no English and started the interview in Russian. '*Gospodin Iyer*,' he started. '*Kogda vee preehali b Moskve?*' I promptly replied, '*Ya preehal shestova Aprelya.*'

To translate this roughly, he asked me when I had arrived in Moscow and I replied that I had arrived on 6 April. This made a huge impact on the dean because he did not expect a new arrival to know any Russian. The rest of the brief interview was conducted through an interpreter. I made it a point to continue learning Russian and would travel in trams to listen to the passengers talking in Russian. Within a few months, I was able to understand everything and even speak in Russian. Some of my office work involved talking to Russian organizations, and I would listen carefully to the interpreter translating our discussions. During the second year of my three-year stay in Moscow, I was able to hold discussions without an interpreter. I was once deputed as the official interpreter to the Defence Minister of India, on a visit to Moscow, for his discussions with his Russian counterpart.

I sent my three children to a Russian School (Number 47) next to my house, and in no time at all Mina, Indu and Param could speak Russian like natives. Indira went on to study Russian at the Honour's level at the Jawaharlal Nehru University in Delhi and has been working as a Russian teacher and interpreter ever since. It is a joke in the family that even now we talk to each other in Russian when we don't want others to know what we are saying. Param had a good opportunity to use his Russian language skill when his daughter, Tara, was playing an ITF tournament in Turkey. Param was Tara's coach-cum-tour-manager, having taken leave from the World Bank in 1997. Tara was playing against a Russian girl and the girl's father was coaching his daughter throughout the match, which is not permitted under ITF rules. Tara won anyway, and as the two girls were shaking hands after the match, Param told the Russian girl's father, in fluent Russian, 'Tough luck, you tried your best to coach her.' As you can imagine, the Russian was hugely embarrassed.

To complete my story, I also learned Marathi, when I spent ten years in Pune after retirement. Now, in my nineties, I continue to learn new languages. I know Tamil and Malayalam fluently. Tamil is my mother tongue and I was born and brought up in Kozhikode. I know Hindi. Now I am learning Kannada and Telugu. How different it is from the time I learned French and Russian. Now when I go on my morning runs I go on YouTube on my mobile and listen to Kannada and Telugu news, commentaries and conversations for an hour. Now I can understand both the languages and converse in them. I also spend some time during the day interacting with Kannada and Telegu teachers online. It is surprising what we can achieve if only we apply ourselves to the task regularly.

I am happy to say that my children also appreciate studying something new, doing something out of the ordinary or celebrating the versatility of our minds. The mind has extraordinary resilience to accept new inputs and learn new skills. Deciding at the age of fifty to study law, Mina, my eldest, enrolled in a law school in Pune and studied law for three years. As she entered the classroom on her first day at the college, all the other students stood up, mistaking her for the lecturer! Of course, soon enough she merged with the class and made some good friends among the students. After passing out with a first class, first rank, she joined a law firm in Chennai. Her work there enabled her to appear before the Supreme Court of

India on three different occasions to plead on two public interest litigation cases on environmental issues.

During my posting in Moscow, I bought a Russian piano and engaged a Russian lady to teach piano to my three children. They were young and quickly picked up the skill. They trained under the teacher for three years and have been playing the piano ever since. My daughters have passed the eighth grade in piano from the Trinity School of Music in England. This is considered the gold standard in piano performance. Indu, in her sixties, continues to play advanced levels of piano music.

As I am in a reminiscent mood, and discussing fitness, let me tell you about the time Param had an unexpected surprise as a young student. He had completed his bachelor's in English literature from St. Stephen's College, Delhi. At the graduation ceremony, the Principal announced a special prize, an award for exemplary behaviour, which went to Param. The Principal told me that Param was conferred this award because he regularly went for a long run every morning in the college campus. Incidentally, this award may also have triggered Param being selected for an exchange scholarship to Davidson College, North Carolina, in 1979.

To move on to my wife. Towards the end of my three-year tenure in Moscow, there was an inter-embassy women's doubles tennis tournament. Our embassy was represented by my wife, Kalyani, and the young daughter of Ambassador Kewal Singh. Now Kalyani was no stranger to tennis. She was the tennis champion at the Queen Mary's College for Women in Chennai, in 1947, and had been playing regularly ever since. After our marriage too, she played regularly, wherever my posting took us in the Air Force. In Jodhpur, it was at the palace of Rao Raja Hanut Singh, where there were four tennis courts. In Srinagar, it was in the Amar Singh Club. She would get the children ready for the evening and entrust them to the care of our old servant Kaba. She would then sit on the handlebar of the bicycle and we would cycle down to the club every evening and play. It was usually doubles and there was an understanding that we did not partner with each other. This would ensure that she won most of the time! There was plenty of tennis when I was training at the Defence Services Staff College in Wellington, Ooty. So Kalyani was in good form when the Moscow inter-embassy tournament took place. Her partner was a beginner but Kalyani's experience took them to the finals. The final was against the Australians, and the match took place in our embassy. The Australian ladies were well-kitted in the typical tennis wear. Kay was in her sari – that is the way she always played tennis. Her partner wore a salwar kameez. It was a closely fought match and the Aussies won in three sets. After the match, they congratulated Kay saying they had expected the match to be an easy affair, seeing the way that the Indian pair was dressed!

After returning from Moscow, I was posted in Chandigarh, where Kay decided to do a teachers' training course to obtain a postgraduate degree in teaching. She joined a regular one-year programme in a city college. As with Mina, she too had the experience of the other students in her class mistaking her for the lecturer and standing up when she entered. Kay was very sensitive and was embarrassed at being dropped off at her college in my newly imported Mercedes-Benz car from Moscow.

She insisted that I drop her a hundred yards before her college campus.

To continue with the tennis saga, I have to fast forward some twenty-five years. I had finished my work at Pondicherry University in 1995 and was ready to move to Chennai, wondering what I should do next. I was sixty-six years old and in no mood to sit quietly at home. Around that time, I read a news item one morning about Ramesh Krishnan, the tennis maestro, planning to start a tennis academy in Chennai. I got hold of his address and shot off a letter offering my services, in an honorary capacity, to help him run the academy. A few days later, all our family members were sitting down for lunch when the telephone rang. No mobiles those days, only landlines. Param picked up the phone and after a second let out a whoop. 'It is Ramesh Krishnan, Appa,' he said. Ramesh was taking me up on my offer and invited me to meet him in Chennai. Thus started a relationship which has lasted to this day. I worked with him to get the Krishnan Tennis Centre started. We had nine clay courts and two synthetic courts. I was the administrator and also coach to young children. Ramanathan Krishnan and Ramesh left the construction of the courts to me. I had a good deal of experience in laying down tennis courts, since I was in the habit of creating a couple of courts at every Air Force base that I was posted to. The KTC, as Ramesh's academy was known, became a premier tennis coaching centre in India thanks to the halo around Ramanathan and Ramesh. Budding young tennis champions migrated to Chennai and trained under the two champions. We had hostel facilities for outstation players. We conducted several tournaments and produced quite a few good players. I spent six years working with Ramesh. Though

I have moved from Chennai, Ramesh and I continue to remain in touch.

Now let us consider the role of the mind in engaging the body. We know that the mind controls the body to the extent that we decide what the body should do at any particular time. We 'will' the legs to stand up or walk or run. When we are agitated, we often will ourselves to calm down, and the heart, in obedience, starts beating slower and slower. These are all manifestations of the mind controlling the body. The body, in turn, can keep the mind busy and calm. For example, when the body is fit, the mind is calm; when we stand on a wobble board and try to balance, we are training the brain to maintain balance. When we jog for a long distance, the mind remains calm and receptive to creative

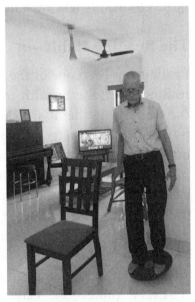

Training the brain to balance using the wobble board

thinking. There is no period in our lives, whatever be our age, when it is not appropriate to take part in physical activities or sports.

I have covered languages, music and sports. There are many other spheres of activity in life, and it is up to us to take advantage of our fitness to pursue any interest of our choice. When we indulge in activities that are not part of our professional life, we enrich our lives. For example, word games are favoured in my family. Scrabble, Boggle

– and now Wordle – are very popular. It is my firm belief that when we participate in such games of skill, it keeps cobwebs away from the brain. Indulge in games that challenge the brain, and the brain will have no time to fall prey to diseases that lie in wait. The brain and the body behave in the same fashion. The brain falls prey to illnesses attracted by its inactivity. Similarly, the body begins to waste away with disuse.

The Reading Habit

Reading has been one of the joys of my life. The joy that reading gives, the breadth of vision that it imparts and the stimulation that it gives to our minds are unmatched by any other learning activity. Just a turn of phrase in a book can launch us into a chain of thought culminating in creative thinking. Literature, fiction, historical treatises, adventure stories and great masterpieces across the centuries – blessed are we who get an opportunity to read even a very small percentage of the available matter. We should rekindle the joy of learning and make special efforts to encourage children to read, and enjoy reading.

Every profession, career or line of work needs physical fitness. We might intuitively feel that cerebral activities do not demand physical fitness. We would be wrong. Viswanathan Anand, the legendary world chess champion, works out regularly in a gym. He says that physical fitness is vital for clear thinking. Regular aerobic exercise keeps the mind alert and does not allow fatigue to set in. Similarly, musicians need a high level of fitness. Sanjay Subrahmanyan, one of the leading Carnatic musicians in India, runs regularly. Fitness brings energy and aura to music, he says.

Yehudi Menuhin, the world-famous violinist, used to say that without physical fitness, he would not have been able to practise every day. And he used to add that without practice, his performance would rapidly plunge. In his own words, 'If I do not practise even one day, I would know the difference. If I do not practise for two days, all my neighbours would gossip, and if I do not practise for three days, why then, the whole world would wonder what happened to my music.' Practice demands fitness of a high order.

When we grow old, good health and a fit body and mind are even more important to continue to enjoy our life. One last word on the relationship between body and mind, and a recipe for getting rid of uneasiness in the mind. Sometimes we find ourselves brooding over some problem or other. It may be a minor matter about some temporary financial difficulty, some unpleasantness in the office or a small family dispute. Whatever it may be, such problems often keep us preoccupied, distracted or even troubled. I too have had my share of such worries. And I am glad to say that I have found a way to get rid of such concerns. I tell myself, 'OK, I have this problem. What is the worst that can happen when this problem evolves? What is the worst situation that this problem can lead to?' The answers to these questions often give me the solution to the problem. Such introspections often solve minor problems. I am talking about small, little problems that crop up in life and not career-threatening situations. If some major crisis crops up, you will need sound advice from people close to you and divine guidance.

There is one exception to the problem-solving technique that I have mentioned. That is when we confront any health issue. We cannot try the same approach and ask ourselves, 'What is the worst that could happen?' Because the worst could be a serious illness. So here the only option is to get it treated by a competent physician.

Sleep

Good sleep is an absolute necessity for good health. Human beings have evolved along with the sidereal rising and setting of the sun, and our sleep is associated with the setting of the sun. Infants sleep almost 20 hours during the 24 hours of the day. Then, while growing up, they settle into a sleep pattern coinciding with the rise and setting of the sun. If we do not get adequate sleep, it will soon affect our health. Therefore, any problems in getting a good night's sleep should be attended to. Generally, good exercise, an early dinner and a good routine before sleeping (whether reading, listening to music or attending to some interesting activity) would ensure good sleep.

The Stress Buster

I conclude this chapter by mentioning the great stress buster – a long walk. A long walk, at any convenient time of the day, would do all kinds of good things to your body and mind. Worries melt away, the mind is at peace and the body has earned an excellent workout. There is no better activity than that walk which blends the body and mind into equilibrium and ensures all-round wellness. At the risk of sounding like a one-trick pony, I do consider running, walking and other aerobic exercises as preventive and protective activities to many of our problems.

SEVEN

Myths and Half-Truths about Fitness

P rint, TV and social media inundate us with information on fitness. We also get advice from friends and colleagues. Unfortunately, much of this information and advice is misleading and some are myths, even if they profess to be based on scientific studies. In this chapter, I examine such myths, half-truths and beliefs to guide you through this barrage of misinformation. I hope this will encourage you to use your common sense in adopting such advice. Let us get started.

Myths about Weight Loss and Gain

Abdominal Exercises Will Reduce Belly Fat

We often hear about the virtue of certain abdominal exercises that are supposed to reduce belly fat – leg raises, sit-ups, oblique crunches, etc. These are all good exercises (and you may perform one or two of them) but they do not contribute to the reduction of belly fat. What they do is strengthen the abdominal muscles. To get rid of belly fat (and indeed fat anywhere in the body), we have to consume fewer calories in a day than we spend that day. Gain and loss of body weight work on a simple principle. To lose weight, our calorie expenditure in a day should be more than the calories that we consume by eating and drinking, during that day.

We spend calories on bodily functions like heartbeat, respiration, digestion, etc., and on physical activities like walking, talking, etc. The total calories spent on these two activities in a day give us our daily calorie expenditure. It is about 2,200 calories a day for a normal person. (It will naturally be more for an active athlete and less for a bedridden person.) Our calorie consumption is what we eat and drink. If we either eat less than 2,200 calories or burn more than 2,200 calories (by a combination of exercise and controlled eating), we will start losing weight. Exercises for stomach muscles will, of course, play their part in reducing belly fat, not directly but to the extent that those stomach exercises contribute towards the total calorie expenditure for the day.

So-Called Magic Foods That Help You to Reduce Your Weight

Be wary of claims that certain foods make you lose weight. Common sense should tell you that there are no such foods. If there were, most of us would be trim and obesity would be a disease of the past. There is no magical food that will help you lose weight. What you eat and drink during a day will decide how many calories you consume. If you reduce your food consumption, you are on your way to weight reduction. Remember that every food item has calories, some more than others. Water is the only exception: it has no calories.

Other Magic Foods: Blood Purifiers

How often do we see advertisements for blood purifiers! We get impressed by the claim that a particular tonic would purify our blood. Who does not want the blood to be pure? But just take a moment to reflect. Is our blood impure? Does it need to be purified? And how does the purification process take place? Yes, indeed the blood constantly needs to be purified because toxic products enter our bloodstream during the process of digestion and our daily activities. For example, during the absorption of proteins, urea and creatinine are introduced into the blood. Both are toxic and need to be removed continuously. This vital job is carried out by the kidneys. The toxic products that we consume like alcohol have to be removed from the blood and that is done by the liver. The kidneys and the liver are the two great blood purifiers. And they have to be kept efficient by normal blood circulation. If you have aerobic fitness, your heart will pump blood to the liver and kidneys, keeping them functioning well. There is no such thing as a blood purifier.

Women and Exercise

Women Become Muscular if They Exercise

I don't know how this myth originated, but it has been around for a long time. Women do not become muscular when they work out with weights or do any other exercises demanding muscular effort. Women have more subcutaneous fat than men and when they exercise their muscles become firmer. But there is no muscle definition; in men, the muscle definition happens because of the absence of fat. For instance, ballerinas or exponents of Indian dances don't look muscular. They are, on the other hand, examples of grace and fluent movement. Incidentally, women need muscular strength as much as men. Most of their activities demand strength;

otherwise, fatigue will set in. All the exercises suggested in chapter 5 are important for women too, and for the same reasons.

Will You Become Fairer if You Drink Milk?

Are you surprised? But believe me, there are a lot of people who think this is true. Some people think it is plausible because milk is white. If we believe in this logic, can you imagine what will happen to our skin, eating, as we do, different colours of food. No, there is no connection between milk and the colour of our skin. Instead, let us talk about the complexion of the skin. The complexion is that quality of the skin which gives the skin its texture, smoothness, shine and beauty. The complexion of our skin is a reflection of our health. When our cardiovascular strength is good, and when the heart pumps out blood to all parts of our body (including the skin), the circulating blood passes on some of its colour to the skin. I have, in an earlier chapter quoted the example of a woman running for several minutes. The subcutaneous blood circulation gives her a dramatic glow. The same thing happens, even without a run, if the blood circulation is efficient – as it will be if you are fit.

This calls to mind a passage from *Pride and Prejudice*, where Mr Darcy was in admiration of the 'brilliancy which exercise had given to Elizabeth's complexion'.

Motherhood and Exercise

There are a lot of myths about motherhood and exercise. After childbearing, mothers are advised to give up competitive sports. This is laughable. There are hundreds of women athletes who have returned to competitive sports after giving birth and won laurels at the highest echelons of sports. Mary Kom, our boxing hero, has won world boxing gold medals after becoming a mother. Kim Clijsters, the tennis legend, won two grand slam tournaments after becoming a mother. My daughter Indu was in her fifties and a mother of three children, when she took part in a veterans ITF tournament in Pattaya, Thailand. Against tough competition from many countries, she reached the final and lost in a closely fought final in three sets to an Australian player. Indu also reached the final of the doubles event. She won the ITF veterans championship held in Sonepat, Haryana, in 2013. Earlier, in 2010, she won a bronze medal in the 400-metre sprint event in the World Veterans Athletics Championship held in Pune. Motherhood, instead of hampering women's fitness, increases their stamina and mental toughness.

Exercise Myths

There are many myths about various techniques that are associated with working out. Here are some of them.

Always Breathe through Your Nose

Many coaches ask their trainees to breathe only through their noses and not through their mouths. As I have mentioned earlier, this is not practical. You won't last long as an athlete if you don't suck in all the air that you need through your nose and mouth. I have seen many athletes in college and school athletics stuffing a handkerchief in their mouth to prevent any accidental breathing through the mouth. Oxygen consumption is the single most important concern during any race and you need to breathe in as much air as you possibly can during a race. There is no ill effect whatsoever in breathing through the mouth during the race. Denying that advantage will not only adversely affect the result of your race but could be dangerous to your health too.

Do Not Drink Water during a Race

This edict is often insisted upon by coaches who are ignorant of elementary physiology. You don't stop to drink water during a sprint, or even during a 10,000-metre race. But for events lasting longer distances like the marathon, it is vital to remain hydrated. Heat exhaustion, and even heatstroke, is an ever-present risk during long-duration events. We can perhaps trace the origin of this myth to coaches who have no patience when young athletes take a water break. But modern sports medicine is very clear about water consumption. Drink as often and as much water as you need during training.

Myths Regarding Training

No Pain, No Gain

This is an oft-repeated slogan of some coaches. It is supposed to encourage the trainees to endure tough training sessions. But science does not support this view. It is not necessary to go through physical pain to achieve fitness or any of its components like strength. In a gym, we go through demanding repetitions, often with heavy weights, but it should not cause any pain. We should not confuse pain with effort. We have to put in the effort to achieve results, but we do not have to endure pain. If a particular workout causes pain, it should be discontinued. Maybe your technique was wrong and you have to get it corrected by the coach. Or maybe you are injured. In aerobic activities, like running, there is no need to go through pain. Effort, yes; discomfort, yes; but no pain. There is a subtle difference between effort and pain. Effort is necessary, but the pain is a warning sign that your technique is wrong.

In the 1960s, Percy Cerutty coached athletes in Australia. Herb Elliot, one of his trainees, won the 1,500-metre race in the 1960 Rome Olympics. Cerutty believed that athletes should go through the pain barrier to achieve success at the highest level. He thought that the energy of an athlete is normally contained in a primary tank in his body. When extra effort is required, as in a race, he or she has to gain access to his or her secondary tank and this can be achieved only through a pain barrier. But Cerutty did not mean physical pain, only extra effort in training.

Sweating during Training

This is another myth that unless you sweat profusely, you have not trained hard enough. Not really! Sweating is a natural body process that helps us get rid of excess body heat when we are engaged in physical activity. But sweating is related to many factors like humidity, ambient temperature, your effort level, etc. It has no relationship to your training benefit. I have run in Washington DC during the winter of 2001. On quite a few occasions, the ground was completely covered with snow. There would be no sweating at all during those runs. The body needs to sweat only when excess heat is generated during an exercise.

The Best Time for Exercise during the Day

I have touched upon this topic earlier in the book, but let me restate the point. Some people say that early morning is the best time for exercise as you are fresh and not tired after a day's work. But others prefer evenings when presumably your worries of the day are over and the exercise routine in the evening helps you get a good sleep. There are yet others who say that it is best to exercise in the office gym during the lunch break because it is convenient.

Let me assure you that the body does not care when you exercise. It only cares whether you exercise. The early morning run is refreshing and gets you ready for the day. You are already ahead of the game, by clocking your workout. Similarly, the evening run removes the strain of the day's work. It matters little when you train. Just do it.

Quick-Fix Fitness

You must have seen ads on YouTube, in fitness-related journals, on TV, and even in newspapers for devices that will help you get fit in just a few days. Some of these ads sell products that claim that by working with those gadgets, you become muscular, lose fat, attain aerobic fitness and derive other fitness goals, all in just a week or two. Well, use your common sense. It is all right to try working out on a machine or elastic band or pulley, so long as you don't pull a muscle using a strange gadget. But reflect for a minute. To become aerobically fit, you need to train the heart, lungs and blood vessels. The training benefit begins to kick in only after working out for at least 20 minutes at a time. It requires several weeks for the body to fully benefit from the training. Above all, remember that fitness is not a destination – it is a way of life. You have to earn fitness every week; you cannot store fitness. So when you buy a gadget to become fit, buy one which you can use for many years.

Specificity

I have come across many aspiring fitness enthusiasts who get disappointed when they cannot play a particular sport, in spite of working on their fitness for weeks and months. Sonavane was a young runner companion of mine. We used to go for long runs when I was stationed in Nagpur in 1985. One Sunday, we started at 5 a.m. and ran a total of 35 kilometres! Normally we used to run 24 to 25 kilometres. It just happened that we were feeling good that Sunday and ran a little more than usual. After bidding goodbye to Sonavane, I reached home. I was exhausted and lay flat on the floor for about 20 minutes. I also had cup after cup of tea. I recovered soon enough but had to rest a good deal during the day. I compared notes with Sonavane later, and he seemed to have had no problems.

Soon after that long run, Sonavane, who was twenty-five years old, was asked to quickly assemble as part of a basketball team to play against a visiting team from the army. He had not practised basketball for several months. Well, within a few minutes into the match, Sonavane was exhausted and had to be replaced. We may wonder why. After all, he was a fit athlete and regularly ran long distances. The answer to this riddle is a phenomenon in sports known as specificity. The body will respond well to an activity to which it is accustomed. The sudden spurt of sprinting and the 'stop and start' technique in basketball are different from the regular cadence of running. The body will have to relearn the movement pattern involved in basketball to be able to do it well and with ease.

Similarly, if you ask a basketball player to do a round of boxing, he will flounder after a few seconds. To be good and fluent in a particular form of physical activity, we need to practise that particular activity. This principle is known as specificity.

Myths (and Reality) Relating to Food

Food is one of the most important joys of life. We all eat till the very end of our lives. Food is a topic of great interest to all of us irrespective of whether we are young athletes, middle-aged seekers of fitness, the elderly or people needing medical help. The print and television media too are obsessed with food. On WhatsApp, Facebook, Twitter, etc., we find an incessant offering of advice on food. Do you want to reduce weight? Easy. Here is the food for you, and you will lose 5 kg in a month! Are you diabetic? No problem. Follow this regime and you will not need any medicine; your sugar level will come down to normal in four weeks. Every conceivable problem, it seems, can be overcome by eating something or avoiding something else. There are pictures of men and women before and after they started on a particular type of food or drink. They show obese people becoming trim and fit within a few weeks of following a particular food regimen. My guess is that the food theme dominates our everyday conversation, with other topics like politics, current affairs and sports coming a distant second.

There must be millions of people who take these messages seriously, and many of them may be experimenting with different types of food.

My daughter Indu takes great interest in studying the effect of food on people. A lifelong vegetarian, she has now started following the vegan diet, which eschews milk, milk products, eggs and all meat. This indeed seems the way forward for the world now.

I too was brought up as a vegetarian. My childhood food was rice, dal and vegetables of a wide variety. I firmly believe consuming such a variety of vegetables had a beneficial effect during the formative years of my childhood.

Even at the age of ninety-two, I relish every meal. I may not eat as much as I used to in the past, but I must confess, it's pretty near as much! I have heard that as we grow older, we eat less, and perhaps do not enjoy eating as much as we did when we were young. But so far, I have never experienced any appreciable lessening of appetite or interest in eating.

So what should we be eating and drinking and how does food affect our lives in general and fitness in particular? Here are my views.

Factors That Make Up Good Food

I shall list the components of good food, with some brief comments on each component.

Variety

A variety of food is important for two reasons. First, variety ensures that we get all the nutrients that we need. What may be missing in one item will be supplied by another. Second, it ensures enjoyment of food and satisfaction with it. I learned one lesson about variety when I was a young officer in the Air Force. I was serving

in the Air Force Flying Academy in Jodhpur. Young
officers are often given what is known as secondary duties,
that is, some work about the station, in addition to our
primary duties. I was thus made the officer in charge of
the airmen's mess. All soldiers in the Air Force get free
food, and if they live in bachelors' quarters, they get to
eat their food in the airmen's mess. My job was to see
that they got good food, prepared in clean and sanitary
kitchens and served in comfortable surroundings. I used
to post the weekly menu on a noticeboard outside the
dining hall. It is usual for visiting dignitaries to inspect
the airmen's mess, as a welfare measure. The then
air vice marshal (AVM) P.C. Lal was on an inspection
visit to Jodhpur Air Base. I was told to receive him at
the airmen's mess and show him around. The first
thing he noticed was the weekly menu sheet on the
noticeboard. The notice stated that the menu was for
11 June to 17 June 1956 (Monday to Sunday). But he
also noticed that the dates had been overwritten over
the previous week's menu (i.e. 4 June to 10 June).
It was obvious that the menu sheet was originally
prepared for the previous week and the same menu
had been repeated, merely changing the dates! As you
can imagine, I was deeply embarrassed. It showed that
I had paid scant attention to the preparation of the
menu and not applied my mind to ensuring variety.
The same AVM Lal eventually became the chief of air
staff and introduced the policy of physical fitness tests
for Air Force personnel, which triggered my interest in
fitness too.

Coming back to variety, after all, it is the spice
of life.

Nutrition

A good diet is one that contains all the elements in appropriate quantities – protein, carbohydrates, fat, minerals, vitamins, to mention a few, are some important components of food. It is not necessary, and not practicable, to include all these components in just one meal. Rather, our aim should be to consume all such elements at least once a week.

Moderation

As we grow older, our metabolic rate becomes slower and we need to eat less food to maintain fitness. Hunger is not a good indicator of how much food we need. A weekly check of our weight is the true test of how much food we are consuming. If your weight remains more or less stationary, you are doing fine. It is so easy to gain weight, and if you are not careful, you can put on several kilos in no time at all. As we know, it is extremely difficult to get rid of the extra weight. Obesity is an ever-lurking disease we need to guard against. Another indicator of whether your food intake is appropriate is your bowel movements. If they are regular, you are on the right track.

So far, I have been treading on safe ground. But now I have to dive headlong into areas that are hotly debated in every country and every scientific and public interest group. What type of food is best for us? Plant-based or animal-based or a combination? I have an advantage when venturing into this controversial debate. As I have mentioned earlier, I was brought up in a vegetarian family and did not even eat eggs till I was in my twenties. Later on in life, I have eaten meat and enjoyed it. Now, in my nineties, I do not eat meat any more but have one egg a day. I do take milk and milk products, but in a limited fashion; for example, I do not drink milk, but use milk for my oats porridge in the morning and three cups of tea a day. I also take yoghurt during meals. My main food consists of rice and a variety of vegetables, nuts, fruits, and seeds (for example, pumpkin seeds added to the morning porridge). I also add a fair amount of cranberries to my morning porridge. When I talk about food and compare vegetarian and non-vegetarian food, I have an open mind and have no prejudice at all.

Let me then say that there is no uniform opinion about vegetarian versus non-vegetarian food in the scientific community, on social media or in forums of public opinion. I have a deep suspicion that the debate about the best kind of food will carry on well into the future, perhaps for several decades. But let me give my thoughts on the subject.

Pros and Cons of a Non-vegetarian Diet

1. **Pros:** good taste; good source of protein; satisfies the urge to eat meat, handed down from our ancestors, who were hunter gatherers
2. **Cons:** chances of toxic decomposition in the intestines during digestion

Pros and Cons of a Vegetarian Diet

1. **Pros:** good taste; variety; a wealth of minerals
2. **Cons:** since some vitamins/minerals are not prevalent in vegetables, we may need some supplements

My conclusion, therefore, is that it is better and safer to stick to a vegetarian diet; or at least a predominantly vegetarian diet, with occasional consumption of meat. As far as the current scientific opinion is concerned, I can only quote some advice that has come from the World Health Organization. Even though this advice has come in the context of COVID-19, the advice is pertinent to nutrition in general.

WHO Advice on Nutrition

1. Limit salt intake
2. Limit sugar intake
3. Limit fat intake
4. Consume enough fibre
5. Drink plenty of water and other fluids
6. Avoid or limit alcohol intake
7. Consume fruits and vegetables
8. Consume whole-grain and starchy food
9. Consume dried fruits, nuts and seeds
10. Consume milk with reduced fat
11. Eggs and fish are good sources of protein

Alcohol

Since October 2020, I have stopped drinking alcohol. That is because I was not able to sleep soundly. I would get up in the middle of the night and toss in bed and it would take me an hour or two to get back to sleep. Once I stopped having a drink, I began to sleep well. I suspect that as we grow older, alcohol might have some adverse effects, especially on sleep. Will I ever have another drink? I don't know.

Conclusion on the Topic of Food

What we eat plays an important part in our well-being. As the saying goes, you are what you eat. The reader must have guessed by now that I am a great devotee of exercise. When the question is asked what is more important for health, exercise or food, my answer is, I don't know. It is such a close call. Let me then conclude this discussion on food on an anecdotal note. In military thinking, there are certain 'principles of war', including the concentration of force and surprise. Napoleon was once asked, 'Who is the general that you would like to have under you to fight an upcoming conflict? Would it be General X, who is a theorist or General Y who is a practical soldier?' Napoleon replied, 'Give me General L, who is lucky.' I could say the same about food, 'Let me choose that food which is lucky for me!'

EIGHT

Managing Disabilities

I do not usually go to a doctor's clinic for consultation. There are two reasons for this. One, I am blessed with a fairly good constitution and do not normally fall ill. Two, a basic fear that the doctor might discover something nasty in my body, which I would rather not know about. But when my right knee began to give me problems, I was forced to go to the hospital. It was sore, and I was not enjoying my daily 2 hours of jogging. Of course, it was not a sudden manifestation. I had known that the knee had developed osteoarthritis, and the condition was gradually getting worse.

Nowadays, all of us have a specialist doctor available for consultation at a moment's notice – the internet! Any minor or major problem with our health, the first thing we do is to look up the symptoms on Google or some other search engine. Doctors caution us against self-diagnosis and self-treatment, but we do it all the time. These days, with the pandemic still roving, who wants to rush to a doctor for every minor problem. So we look up the symptoms on the internet. The only problem is, more often than not, our symptoms could mean any number of maladies starting from a common cold to the most dangerous lung ailment. But certain conditions, like arthritis of the knee, are susceptible to self-study. I had a series of X-rays taken of my right knee, over the years, and they showed a steady narrowing of the space between the two major bones of the upper and lower leg, at the knee joint. Normally, there is a thick, soft tissue called the meniscus between the two bones. It is a cartilage that acts as a lubricant between the bones so that there is no discomfort when the bones move. But this cartilage gets worn and becomes thinner and thinner, until, as in my case, there is nothing between the two bones to provide lubrication.

Medical science does not know why this happens. It generally occurs in middle age, and age is cited as a reason for it. Google says that most people above fifty years develop this problem. I have been suffering from it for more than twenty-five years. Over those years, I have consulted several orthopaedic surgeons and shown them the X-rays taken periodically. There has been steady wear and tear on the cushioning. The condition is not curable, but certain countermeasures help to mitigate the problem. These include strengthening the muscles surrounding the knee (the muscles of the upper and lower leg), losing weight, stretching often and continuing to use the leg regularly.

I have been following the advice religiously and regularly work out in the gym, paying particular attention to strengthening my upper and lower parts of the leg. This is why I am still able to run without a break.

I do my best to keep my weight to a minimum. I stretch regularly and, of course, I run every day for at least 2 hours.

Coming back to my visit to the hospital. This was in early 2020, just before the COVID-19 pandemic began. The surgeon at the Air Force Command Hospital in Bangalore asked me to meet him at the orthopaedic ward, where he was on a round. He looked at the latest X-ray reports and said to me, 'Sir, you are ninety years old!' I admitted to the crime. 'Do you know that your knee is bone to bone? You should be in a wheelchair. I am surprised you are walking.'

I told him that I was also running every day for 2 hours. He was aghast to hear that and said what I needed was a knee replacement. But because of my advanced age, it would not be advisable to undergo surgery. 'In your case, sir, I would suggest underwater exercises for the leg. You could also try a stationary bike for exercise.'

If that doctor had taken an extra 2 minutes out of his busy schedule, he might have noticed the muscular strength still noticeable in my legs, the result of a regular, devoted strength training schedule that I have been following for decades. Of course, he didn't know about the thousands of kilometres that I have run. After the visit, I have run close to another 5,000 kilometres and my knees are no worse than before! I have also lost 2 kg of weight since then, and that has helped me feel light when I jog. My advice, therefore, to those of you who suffer from osteoarthritis of the knee is continue to run or walk as usual, get rid of the extra weight and strengthen your leg muscles regularly in the gym or at home with home gym equipment.

Losing weight is particularly important. When you run, you land heavily on your feet, and the knees take much of the load. Every kilo of weight that you lose will help you land with 4 kg less weight.

As we advance in age, we are prone to various kinds of disabilities. They creep in unnoticed. It is important to realize that old age is not a disease just as infancy is not one. Each stage of life presents its challenges, and we need to be aware of them and deal with them in a practical, common sense-driven and science-assisted way. Consult a paediatrician if it is a child-related medical problem and a gerontologist if it is about old age. Let us now look at the problems that we often face when we grow old. I have already dealt with osteoarthritis.

Problems with Vision

The health of our eyes often deteriorates as we grow older. One of the main reasons for this is what is known as age-related macular degeneration (AMD), brought on by poor retinal blood circulation. Regular aerobic exercise can help in warding off this disease. Glaucoma, another progressive disease of the eye, is due to an increase in intraocular pressure. There is evidence that this too can be prevented by aerobic exercise. Cataract has no direct connection with blood circulation and needs to be cured through surgery and implantation of artificial lenses.

Dental and Ear-Related Problems

If I have given an impression that all age-related problems can be warded off by aerobic exercise and strength training, it is time to disabuse you of this notion. Many conditions develop as we advance in age. Our teeth, for example, need attention. Dental health is important for all of us. Poor dental hygiene can have serious consequences on our health. It can lead to the infection spreading to our organs. It is important to take good care of our teeth by daily cleaning, flossing and regular visits to the dentist.

Similarly, loss of hearing affects many people. There may be many reasons for this and you need to consult an ENT surgeon to help you with these conditions.

Cervical Spondylosis

As we grow older, our spine undergoes degenerative changes. The space between the spinal discs tends to shrink and we may experience discomfort or pain. Naturally, we have to consult specialists. They often prescribe physiotherapy to keep the problem under control. Many years ago, a physician told me about the importance of physiotherapy. But at that time, I did not fully appreciate its significance. But now, I recognize that it is an effective, indispensable therapy that can be done at home, once you have learned the technique.

I have been diagnosed with cervical spondylosis and was prescribed physiotherapy exercises. I have been doing these exercises regularly, and I am glad to say that I have never again experienced any pain or discomfort. Some of these exercises require resistance bands, which usually come in a set of three or four different coloured, flexible bands. They are extremely useful not only for cervical exercises but also for strengthening shoulder and hand muscles. Exercises using resistance bands are very easy to do and you can easily learn how to use them by reading the literature supplied with the bands, or by watching exercises using resistance bands on YouTube.

Skin Problems

The skin is the biggest organ in the body. Healthy skin ensures a good defence mechanism against the ever-present and lingering pathogens waiting to enter our bodies. Healthy skin reflects a healthy body. As we grow old, the skin tends to wrinkle and becomes dry. The connective tissues tend to become weak and rupture, producing subcutaneous bleeding. Specialists call it senile purpura. It is wise to apply oil to the skin at least once a week to keep the skin pliant and healthy. Coconut oil or any vegetable oil is good for this purpose. It is important to realize the beneficial effect of applying oil on the skin. In Kozhikode, we knew an ayurvedic doctor, Chandu Vaidyar. He once told us that oil preserves the body in many unknown ways. He used to say, 'Oil can even preserve dead bodies (embalming), what to say of living beings!'

Prevention of Exercise-Related Injuries

Enthusiastic pursuit of running, walking or other aerobic activities sometimes causes injuries. They are often a result of overtraining. We need to guard against them. The body gives out various signals when you overtrain. Headache, colds, lack of enthusiasm to train and tiredness which doesn't go away after rest are some of the symptoms of overtraining.

My Encounter with the Consequences of Overtraining

When I was just short of ninety years, I used to frequent a gym called Global Wings in north Bangalore and work out there six days a week, in the mornings, after my 2.5-hour run. One day, while I was doing leg extension exercises, I suddenly felt extremely tired. I had no enthusiasm to continue. I did not even feel like finishing the set I was doing. I just collected my kit and went home. I did not know what had hit me. Later in the day, I realized that

I was a victim of overtraining. I had been pounding the ground, working out in the gym relentlessly, with just a Sunday off from the gym and no break at all from my runs. It was time to unwind and take a break. And that is what I did. I stopped all fitness-related activities. It took me a whole week to recover and get back the enthusiasm for training. We need to be constantly on guard against overtraining. In my case, it was luckily only a week's break, but I have heard of colleagues who felt jaded for several weeks.

Pain is another sign that you are overtraining. Pay heed to pain and cut back on training. Lack of flexibility, especially in the hamstrings, can cause pain in the knee or lower leg. Make sure that you stretch those muscles regularly.

A stitch is a sudden pain on either side of your lower rib cage. It sometimes comes on when you start a run or walk. It is not a serious condition, but it can be painful enough to stop you from running. It is a sign that you have not warmed up. Bend forward and press the affected area with your palms. Generally, there will be quick relief.

You may also experience cramps while you are walking or running. Stop your activity and stretch the muscle that has cramped. For example, if your hamstring muscles have cramped, stand up and try to bend and touch your toes. If the quadricep has cramped, bend your knees. These are simple measures and it is good to be aware of them.

Healthy Eating

Even though I have discussed food as a factor in keeping fit, here is a quick relook at our eating habits as a preventive measure to ill health. A doctor once told me that while we are not much concerned about general illness, we get concerned when it comes to stomach-related problems. So while we may not pay as much attention to chest pain, we are immediately worried by a stomach ache. It may be that chest pain is a more serious health issue, but what grabs our attention is the stomach-related problem. We can take some simple steps to reduce the chances of a stomach-related problem.

Avoid Overeating

It is easy to give this advice, but very difficult to follow. So I am going to suggest two approaches to curtail overeating. The first one is to get up from the dining table when you know that you can eat some more. This is easier said than done. My brother-in-law once told me with a straight face, 'Place both your palms on the dining table, and press them both down hard enough to straighten your elbow, making you stand up. Then walk away from the dining table. But,' he added, 'this exercise has to be performed when you are halfway through your meal.' Easy for him to make fun of me, but the greed for eating is always lurking. I have come across a few people who do not like food. They come from all walks of life. For instance, Ashwathayya, a taxi driver in Bangalore keeps a bottle of water and no other food item in his car. He eats two rotis in the morning and nothing else till night. Lean, fit and hardy, he is. If you are in that mould, good luck to you. Lesser mortals like me have to depend upon extra exercise to keep our weight under control. There are a few methods of counteracting the tendency to overeat. Eat plenty of fibre and other low-calorie food so that your stomach is satiated and you have no craving to eat any

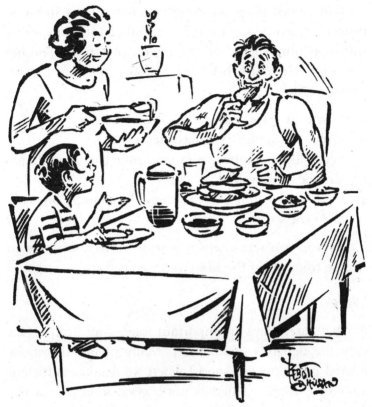

Exercising does not give you the licence to overeat!

more. Fibre should be an important part of your food, in its own right. Many vital functions are performed by fibre in the course of digestion:

1. Fibre bulks up the stool for easy defecation.
2. Fibre lubricates the bowel for easy passage of nutrients and helps in their absorption.
3. Fibre induces satiation and prevents overeating.
4. Fibre also increases peristalsis (the muscular contractions that move food through the bowels) and relieves the feeling of fullness of the stomach.

Gut health plays an important part in our immune system's response to infections, and therefore consuming sufficient fibre should be the main concern in planning our food. Here is a brief list of foods that are a good source of fibre:

1. Grains like rice, wheat, oats
2. Fruits like apples, bananas, guava
3. Seeds like pumpkin seeds, and nuts like groundnuts, almonds and walnut
4. Potatoes, green leafy vegetables like spinach, broccoli, and cabbage

As you can see, there is a wide variety of foods to choose from to get the fibre that we need.

Water

Finally, water plays an important role in our health. Our very life depends upon water. Many of our digestion-related problems get solved when we drink a sufficient amount of water. Thirst is not a good indicator of our requirement for water. It is, therefore, wise to drink water periodically. You should drink plain water rather than beverages that contain sugar and salt. These beverages tend to be hypertonic, that is, they demand more water from our cells for neutralization, depleting our water store.

Accidents

An accident, by its very definition, is something that happens when we least expect it. It has happened to most of us. I met with an accident when I was eighty-seven years old. I had read that it is good to run backwards for 5 minutes after a long run. It is supposed to help balance the load on the legs. So after finishing my daily run, I would spend a few minutes jogging backwards. I never had any problems except one day when I tripped and fell. My right wrist took the load and was fractured. The orthopaedic surgeon in the hospital examined the wrist and confirmed that I had a fracture. He said I would need a cast for six weeks. So began my recovery. Luckily, I could run with the cast.

However, I was not lucky with my convalescence. Occasionally, such injuries culminate into a nasty condition known as chronic regional pain syndrome. The condition happens due to a malfunction of the nerves of the hand. It often causes unbearable pain, as if the hand has been immersed in a burning fluid. My problem was detected early and treated at AIIMS, Delhi. The doctor would greet me with a firm handshake, which would send jolts of pain in my fractured wrist. He explained that he did this to check the degree of pain. As part of the medicines for tissue recovery, he prescribed vitamin C. I was hesitant as I used to take oranges regularly. My doctor said I could skip the vitamins if I had a hundred oranges a day!

Running backwards demands extra care because we don't know what is behind us. Similarly, in our everyday lives, we need to be extra careful in areas in our houses where there are chances of slipping and falling. The bathroom is a typical example. It is a good idea to install one or two bars or handholds that we can grasp when negotiating slippery areas.

Tonics for the Mind

Young or not so young, there are times in our daily routine when we feel lethargic, bored, stale, demotivated or just lacking in enthusiasm. If it is temporary, we can soon spring back to an active life. But if one or two of these manifestations persist, you must attend to them because they can affect your quality of work and productivity. There are many avenues to engage your mind – music, reading, pets, yoga and sports – and you have to choose what works best for you. Then there is the ultimate tool of today, the internet. With just a touch of the finger, you are transported to a world of activities, information and entertainment. And remember, there is always that ultimate stress buster, a long walk.

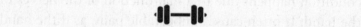

NINE

Occupational Hazards of the Fitness Seeker

While it is fun to go out on a long jog or walk, we have to be on guard against various kinds of dangers that we might encounter. Based on my experience, let me lay out before you what hazards you may run into while out on a running session.

Buffaloes

First and foremost I would like to give an account of an improbable incident that happened to me. It was in 1982. I was in great running form. As usual, I was out running at 5 a.m. It was pitch-dark. As I was running down the Seminary Hills, with hardly a care in the world, I banged headlong into something hard like a wall. I could have sworn that there was nothing in front of me, as I was running in the middle of the road. The impact blew the breath out of my chest. And suddenly I realized that I had run into a buffalo! I don't know who was more surprised, the buffalo or I. One moment it was standing on the road, chewing the cud or whatever buffaloes do early in the morning, and the next, this heavy collision. I did not pause to apologize!

Dogs

Dogs are lovely animals. We once had a pet dog named
Bondy. The fun and joy that we had when Bondy was
alive will fill a chapter. But I am now talking about street
dogs. They are very suspicious of runners. A runner, in
their mind, is an intruder into their territory and needs
to be chased away. I have developed a strategy to deal
with them. If they are far away and start growling, I try
to avoid looking at them and jog on. I have heard that
barking dogs seldom bite. The crucial word here, however,

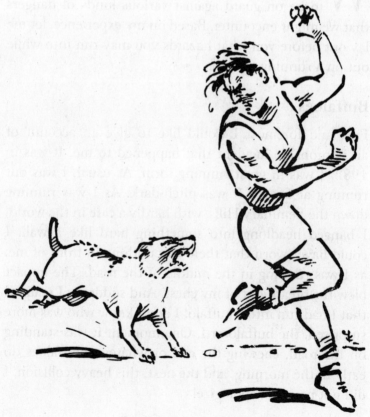

Beware of street dogs!

is 'seldom'. I don't want to be the exception. So if they start barking and come closer, I take steps. I pick up a stone. Even if there are no stones, I pretend to pick up one. Normally, the dog gets the message and backs off. But if the dog persists in barking and approaches me, I let out a blood-curdling yell that has surprised many a dog.

But once I was put in a position of immense danger. I was commanding an Air Force unit in Chakeri, Kanpur, in 1980. I was running on the Kanpur–Allahabad highway and had run about 6 kilometres when I almost collided with a huge dog. It was so near that there was no time to execute my stone-picking manoeuvre. There was a small village nearby and the dog must have belonged to one of the villagers. Such dogs are very dangerous because they think that they are saving the village from criminals. I was almost paralysed with fear. People say that dogs can smell fear. It must have smelt mine because it was barking ferociously. As I was resigning myself to my imminent fate, an old man came by with a stick in his hand. He saw my plight and shouted at the dog, waving his stick. The dog got the message and backed off.

I was not so lucky when I had my second encounter with a dog. This was in 1996. Ramesh Krishnan and I were running in front of the MCC cricket ground towards the Marina Beach. It was our Sunday morning routine. That day, we had just started our run when a dog came from behind me and bit me on my left ankle. There was a sharp pain before I realized that I had been bitten. I asked Ramesh to carry on with his run and quickly returned to the MCC ground. I went straight to the washroom and kept the wound under the water for a minute or two. It is important to wash away as much of the toxin as possible with running water. It is also vital to start taking a course of anti-rabies injections, starting from the day of the bite. And that is what I did.

To continue with my saga with dogs, the last time I had to deal with a street dog was in 2012 in Chennai. I was eighty-three years old then and, of course, doing my inexorable early morning run when a bunch of street dogs suddenly pounced on me from nowhere. There were three or four of them. All huge ones, fondly fed by shopkeepers nearby. As usual, they thought they were protecting their territory. The leader among them was particularly ferocious. It was very early in the morning and no help was at hand. I was carrying my water bottle in a bag and aimed a heavy blow at the leader's snout with my bag. It immediately withdrew and the other dogs followed suit. I had to write off my bag and the water bottle because they had got soiled. A small price to pay I thought.

To avoid the menace of dogs, you must choose a park or a track or a school compound for your workout. If you have to run on the roads, try to do it during daylight hours when there is less chance of a dog chasing you. For some strange reason, if there are two of you running, dogs generally stay away from you.

Birds

Yes, birds can be a hazard too. I used to run in the National Stadium in Delhi. The stadium has a 400-metre track and trees surrounding the ground, which add to the charm of the place. The only problem was that eagles fly in the sky above the stadium. I often noticed them flying lower and lower, and hovering above me. Perhaps they mistook me for a fluffy, slow-moving bird. Once, an eagle came within touching distance of my head and I got the message. From then onward, I started wearing a cap to cover my head and the eagles never troubled me after that.

But unfortunately, crows are more intelligent than eagles. They don't like humans running around close to their nests. They suspect evil intentions on their eggs and fledglings. Once I was running near a tree where a crow had built a nest. The crow flew straight into my head, deliberately. Luckily, I was wearing a cap and was not injured. But I got the message and avoided that area. However, I was not lucky when a similar thing happened about seven years ago. I was running in a shady area. There were plenty of trees there, and, you guessed it, there were crows, and it was nesting time. I was not wearing any headgear and a crow flew into the top of my head and scraped my scalp with its beak. There was a slight bleed and so I was back to the hospital for another course of anti-rabies injection. So be alert when you are working out near trees. Look out for birds that might be hovering.

Snakes

Snakes don't attack us unless we trample on them. I have had close encounters with snakes on several occasions, mainly because I run between four and six in the morning. That is the time when snakes are active, looking out for prey. The only thing we can do to guard against them is to avoid bushy or stony areas and stick to well-lit places. Whenever I had to go through a rough patch of ground, I used to lift my knees and run. Good training for a fast run!

Other animals might harm you, especially if you are running alone and in a lonely, wild area. Once I had read a newspaper report of a mountain lion attacking and badly injuring a woman runner in the hillocks in California. That was too tragic. As runners, we should be aware of our surroundings and careful about when and where we run.

Losing One's Way

I have never lost my way while running in strange places because I make it a point to orient myself when in an unknown area. But when Param was on an exchange scholarship to Davidson College in North Carolina, he set out on a run with a friend, Tim, one evening. They ran south towards Charlotte, a big city, some 30 kilometres south of Davidson. After running 8 kilometres, they had to run through a diversion and got lost. It started raining and no one could be sighted who could help them. Eventually, they spotted a lady waiting at a bus stop. They jogged up to her and asked whether they were on the right road to Davidson College. The lady burst out laughing, as she replied, 'You guys are on the right road to the loony bin.' As the poor youngsters turned away, hurt and confused, the woman continued to laugh heartily.

Weather and Other Elements

Weather conditions can affect the quality of our workouts. When it is pleasant, with a gentle breeze blowing on our face, we are consumed with the joy of running, with no care in our mind. But heat, humidity, air pollution and many such adverse conditions can overwhelm us as we go about with our daily routine. What can be done about them? We should respect the various manifestations of nature. In our daily workouts, we should accept the weather presented to us, and tailor our exercise to flow with the conditions.

Heat

Heat can adversely affect us when we venture out in the open. As we walk or run, heat starts building up in our bodies. We sweat to get rid of the heat. This is vital for our well-being. Extreme heat can cause heat exhaustion and heatstroke, especially when it is humid. Humidity reduces the effect of sweating. This was demonstrated to us a few years ago. I was escorting my grandson Venkat, as he was taking part in the professional tennis circuit in India. Madurai, in Tamil Nadu, was the final leg of the circuit. It was April and the temperature in Madurai was about 38 degrees Celsius. It was humid too. The match started at 11 a.m. Venkat was by then fully acclimatized to the weather because he had been playing tournaments during the previous few weeks, under similar conditions. The match in Madurai was the quarter-final and went to three sets. Soon after the match, Venkat looked extremely exhausted. His skin was warm to the touch. We rushed him to a hospital nearby. It was a case of heat exhaustion, and he was put on drips. He recovered in about half an hour and the danger had passed. The attending doctor said that it could easily have progressed to heatstroke, which is a medical emergency. If a very fit, trained and acclimatized young man can be hit by heat, it can happen to any one of us.

Most of us do not compete in professional sports. We try to keep fit by doing physical training at our own time, place and convenience. We can avoid the hot periods of the day. We can choose shady areas. At the worst, we can even avoid working out on days that present severe adverse weather. Under normal summer conditions, we should make sure that we are well hydrated. Always carry a water bottle with you when out for a walk or a run. And take frequent sips of water even if you are not thirsty.

Cold Weather

Cold weather is not so difficult to negotiate unless it is extremely cold. Warm-up is always a good idea before we start on a run. But in extremely cold weather, the warm-up assumes greater importance. We should not present ourselves to extremely cold temperatures because that puts us at the risk of developing hypothermia or very low body temperature. Wear a cap because a major portion of heat loss occurs through the head. If you are running in Ladakh or some such cold areas in winter, you have to dress appropriately and warm up indoors before venturing out.

If you are in an area where there is snowfall, you need to take care that you run or walk in a place where there are people.

Rain

Running in the rain can be great fun, but if the rain is accompanied by lightning, beware! If lightning strikes suddenly, try to move to the nearest building. If there is no building nearby, get into a car, or failing that, stay away from trees. Trees attract lightning bolts.

Altitude

I have touched upon altitude before in this book when talking about getting acclimatized. We should not take chances with height, heat and other elements. If you are well acclimatized, they will not harm you. If you are not, you could be hard hit by them. During the Mexico Olympics in 1968, long-distance runners could not perform anywhere near their potential because Mexico City is at an altitude of 2,240 metres. At that height, there would be a great reduction in performance, unless we get acclimatized.

Pollution

I started wearing a mask much before the advent of COVID-19. I used to live in Delhi with Param from 2016 to 2020. Delhi was and perhaps still is the most polluted city in India. The air quality index (AQI) often reaches the 'hazardous' level. Citizens who go about their work may not notice the adverse effect of air pollution on a day-to-day basis, but it is bound to affect their health in the long run. Runners can notice the toll that toxic air takes on their lungs. We can feel the lungs getting fatigued during the latter part of the run.

A mask was not considered necessary about a decade ago because of a lack of awareness about the harm air pollution causes to our lungs. Running in the streets always involves breathing the air toxified by the exhaust fumes of motor vehicles. But that is the price we have to pay for living in cities. An N95 mask is considered the gold standard for masks, whether to guard against dust or viruses.

Middle-Aged Runners and Children

Children are certainly not a hazard to runners. But sometimes, their innocent pranks can affect our equanimity. As mentioned earlier, I used to run on the banks of the river Ganga in Kanpur. The area used to be completely deserted. One day, while I was running, a boy about eight or nine years old appeared on top of the steps leading down to the banks of the river. He watched me running for some time and then started shouting '*chikkani, chikkani*', pointing at me. I did not know what it meant, but knew it was nothing complimentary. I ignored it of course and kept doing my exercise. The next day, I checked up with a colleague who was a native Hindi speaker. He said *chikkani* meant a 'shameless person'! The poor boy, in his innocence, perhaps thought an elderly person should be sitting at home with a blanket around him. It is up to us runners to understand children's behaviour in its context.

But another encounter I had with children was not so harmless. It was in Nagpur. I was out running one evening. It was getting dark and there was no one in the Gondwana Hills. Suddenly, a group of young children appeared from a hut. I was running up and down a gradient, happy with my thoughts, when a stone fell near me. I looked up and saw one or two children picking up stones and aiming them at me. They must have thought that I was mad, and children of that age like to tease mad people. Discretion being the better part of valour, I quietly left that spot in a hurry and was able to escape any harm.

A middle-aged runner has to be canny and learn to live in the society in which he finds himself. Hopefully, children who mock and try to harm people will grow up to understand that middle age demands exercise to keep fit.

Let me not give the impression that we have to be on the lookout for hazards that might be in store for us. On the contrary, working out in the open is a highly exhilarating activity. We look forward to our getting out and enjoying ourselves. And that is how it should be.

TEN

An Invitation to the Fitness Club
(Which You Cannot Afford to Refuse)

Social media has hundreds of articles and learned treatises on the subject of health. It would be accurate to say that the overwhelming weight of advice boils down to two pieces of advice:

1. Regular exercise is essential to good health
2. Keeping the brain active is essential for mental well-being

I am going to illustrate, with examples from my life, how you can achieve both these goals. It does not take an extraordinary effort to be fit. The effort required can be woven into your daily life, without making any dramatic changes.

An Emergency in the Hospital

Let me start with an incident that took place when I was serving in Nagpur. My mother-in-law was admitted to the government hospital for emergency surgery for an obstruction in the intestines. She was recovering in the hospital and Kay was with her. One Sunday, I offered to relieve my wife from hospital duties for a few hours. A room next to my mother-in-law's room was empty and I decided to take rest there as I had run 15 kilometres in the morning and was rather sleepy.

I also thought that in case I was needed, I would be right next door. I don't know how long I slept, but when I woke up, I found a nurse measuring my temperature. I tried to gesture to her that I was not a patient, but she said, 'Relax, sir, this will only take a minute.' She also measured my pulse and suddenly rushed out of the room, saying, 'Sir, I will be back in a minute.' The door flung open and two doctors were ushered in by the nurse. 'The pulse is forty-three, sir,' exclaimed the nurse. The senior doctor asked me, 'How are you feeling, sir.' I told them that I was not a patient but had come to keep an eye on the patient next door. When I told the doctor that I was a long-distance runner, he immediately understood the reason for the low pulse rate and told the nurse not to worry about me. Sometimes you have to pay a price for being fit!

I have run 1,20,000 kilometres! You may wonder why I consider my running total of 1,20,000 kilometres such a big deal. Let me put it in context. Let us compare that mileage with other long-distance runners (all unknown to me of course). Some people have run many marathons. But remember, a marathon is only 42 kilometres, and a thousand marathons are only 42,000 kilometres. Others run ultra-long distances of 150 or 300 or even 500 kilometres. Again, even a hundred of those 500 kilometres will only total 50,000 kilometres. Of course these runners all train, in addition to racing. Even giving them the same amount of mileage for training, they don't approach anywhere near my mileage. Mine is a result of an everyday effort, averaging 8 kilometres a day. That is what I have been doing these past forty-five years. It is the steady, inexorable daily pounding of the roads that has made me what I am today. It is this experience that I want to call upon when I invite you to have a fresh look at your need for fitness. I argue that (a) you can start a fitness programme at any age, and (b) it can be achieved by adjusting or modifying your daily life slightly.

A Proactive Approach to Fitness

Whatever your age, to become fit, to be in with a chance to lead a healthy, long life, is a rightful and achievable ambition. As has been repeatedly and amply brought out in the earlier chapters, you can start at any age, and become fit in no time at all. Whether you are in your forties, fifties, sixties, seventies, eighties or even nineties, whether you are a man or a woman, whatever your earlier lifestyle, I am offering you this chance to get back to sturdy health and have a shot at living a long life. But the effort needs to be proactive. That is, if you say to yourself, 'I am going to go out and do some walking or jogging or cycling, and let me see what happens,' it is not going to work. There are too many uncertainties in life, and your good intentions are not enough to deal with those uncertainties. You need a structured approach.

Setting Targets

Management schools play a game where students are gathered in groups of ten and each student is asked to throw a tennis ball into a basket. The basket is placed in a corner of the room, but the students are not told from where to throw the ball. Some stand near the basket and throw the ball easily into the basket. While others stand far away and try to throw the ball into the basket with obviously poor outcomes. Their attitude is that they can't be blamed for the failure because they had set themselves a difficult task. But a few stand at a distance of 3 metres or so from the basket. They have an even chance of putting the ball inside. They choose a demanding but achievable target. So should you, when approaching fitness.

As mentioned earlier, you can achieve total fitness in three months even if you have never exercised before. This statement is made based on my experience. Without any interest or experience in gaining fitness, I was catapulted from an ordinary middle-aged person into a fit athlete within just three months. And because of the enthusiasm I gained by looking at my fitness and energy levels, I was able to maintain that fitness, and even build on it during the past forty-five years. And so can every one of you. Instead of looking at the next three months, take two weeks of fitness-related activities at a time. Whatever your choice of exercise, go for it with the conviction that you are going to give it all your enthusiasm. Four weeks may seem too long for you to follow a strict regime. So, choose two weeks. There is a ring of regularity or purpose or pattern to two weeks. This, then, is your litmus test. If you can stick to your two weeks of exercise, you have taken a huge step forward. Six weeks is all it takes for your regimen to start showing results. Your breathing rate will be slower, you will feel lighter and fitter and eventually complete 1-hour exercise with ease and even with comfort. And then, all of a sudden, you seem to have the excitement of going ahead with the regime for another six weeks and that makes it three months. You are there. You have arrived. You are a different person altogether!

Short Cuts to Fitness

Don't be misled by advertisements that claim that you can be fit without doing any hard exercise. There are plenty of such claims in social media, TV ads and even in newspapers. 'Wear this belt for ten days and you will lose 2 kilos,' says one ad. 'Lose weight by sweating,' says another ad. 'Wear this jacket for one hour, and you sweat out your extra kilos,' screams another. There is no such shortcut to losing weight or becoming fit. In any case, fitness is not a two-week enterprise – it is a lifelong journey.

We should use our God-given common sense and make decisions based on logic. The main requirement for becoming fit is a healthy heart. And you make the heart healthy simply by making it work hard.

The Human Heart

Our heart, a fist-sized organ, works 24 hours a day, throughout our lives, from birth to death, without a single second of rest. It pumps 7,000 to 8,000 litres of blood in a single day and nurtures all the organs and cells in our body. And the great wonder is that despite performing such an astonishing task, it becomes stronger by working harder. Our body consists of many systems – the nervous system, the respiratory system, the digestive system, etc. – but the one system that remains rugged even in later life is the cardiovascular system. Nature intended it to be strong because our life depends on it. We may become short of hearing and our eyes may not remain sharp, but we need to breathe and we need blood circulation, and that is what the cardiovascular system does. And the mantra to keep it strong is exercise.

Incidentally, apart from the hospital incident where a nurse created an emergency-like situation, there was another occasion when my physiology was mistaken for a cardiac affliction. I was serving in Kanpur, in the Chakeri Air Force Complex, in 1980. I was at the height of my running abilities. I used to go to a maidan near the Air Force Station every morning and run around the track for about 2 hours. There were a few factories in that area and they used to spew smoke into the atmosphere. Those days, there was not much awareness of AQI and atmospheric pollution. It never occurred to me to wear a mask, especially when running. After a few days of running there, I started getting a feeling of congestion in my chest. I went to a nearby physician and he asked for a chest X-ray. The radiologist told me that I might be having a condition known as left ventricular hypertrophy or an enlarged left ventricle of the heart. In matters medical, I often seek a second opinion. So I went to a senior heart specialist and showed him the X-ray report. I also told him about my lifestyle and how I run regularly. He examined me, listened to my running history and concluded that there was nothing wrong with me. He told me that the left ventricle of my heart had expanded so that I could accommodate a larger volume of blood. It is, of course, hypertrophy, but very much benign. It is sometimes referred to as an athlete's heart. My heart pumps a larger quantity of blood than a normal person's, and it helps me to run more efficiently. As for my chest congestion, he suggested that I wear a mask when I ran to avoid the ambient pollution. This is what I did. At the risk of repeating myself, when you consult a doctor, always mention your lifestyle and what type of fitness training you are undergoing.

How about People Who Can't Spare the Time?

I expect that there will be people who may not be able to devote 1 hour a day to fitness. It may be due to work pressure, family commitments or frequent travel. To those people, I would like to offer an alternative route to fitness. Nothing is perfect in this world and we have to make do with what we have. It need not be all or nothing in the realm of fitness. Dr Morehouse, a famous doctor, had argued that all it takes to remain fit is as little as 15 minutes of simple exercises in a day. And the exercises he suggested were free hand exercises like touching your toes, bending forward, backward and sideways, Stretching one hand over the head towards the other side and a bit of walking. He claimed that these simple everyday exercises can help a person remain fit. Most of his contemporary doctors were sceptical about his claims. According to them, a minimum of 4 or 5 hours of exercise needs to be devoted a week to remain fit. But Dr Morehouse's theory attracted many adherents, and they all started exercising. And having started, they were hooked on to a life of exercise. So can you. Start with a small workout and see where it takes you.

COVID-19 and the Way Forward

In our quest for fitness, we need to guard against falling ill. During the COVID-19 pandemic that devastated the world in 2020 and is only now beginning to show signs of abating somewhat, I, like countless others, watched helplessly as the disease unfolded, spreading misery. I have been studying the gradual build-up of reliable theories regarding the many variants of the virus, their characteristics, their method of infection, their typical manifestation on the affected and the post-recovery convalescence. As the theories are still evolving, we have to wait to understand fully the present and likely future scenarios. Let me try to put in a nutshell the available advice on prevention and post-recovery convalescence.

I have so far been able to ward off the disease. I have been something of an escape artist, literally dodging it in the nick of time. I was living in Bangalore during the spread of the disease for the past two years with my daughter Indu. I was due for my second vaccination when Indu and her husband Jayaraman were found COVID-19 positive. Luckily, my other daughter, Mina, had just shifted her residence from Chennai to Bangalore and had taken up a flat in the same society where I lived. I quickly shifted to Mina's residence. This was in May 2021, when the second wave, Delta, was raging. I duly got my second vaccination and escaped the infection then. In February 2022, Mina developed fever and the RT-PCR test came positive. I again did my dodging act and went back to Indu's house. Everyone may not be as lucky as me, but what all of us can do is try our best by taking precautions.

Precautions against COVID-19

Everyone knows what these precautions are. Wear a good mask whenever going out, and even in your house if people are coming to visit you. When in doubt, wear a double mask. Make sure that your family members also wear masks. I wear a mask at home whenever my children or grandchildren visit. A mask prevents a fistful of the virus from entering our breathing airways. A certain minimum viral load is required for the disease to take hold in your body. Surely, we can all take this elementary and primary precaution to guard against infection!

Apart from wearing a mask, keep a hand sanitizer handy and clean your palms whenever you handle any item, whether the buttons in the elevator or any other object. Observe social distancing everywhere. These are all small adjustments but they can save you from an infection. One reason I have not been infected is that I wear a mask most of the time at home, and of course every time I go out including when I go out to jog every morning. The virus, after all, enters your body mainly through your nose or mouth, and if you cover them effectively with a good mask, there are very few chances of your getting infected. This also applies to whichever new variant of the virus emerges.

Another essential protection against COVID-19 is to get vaccinated. Every bit of scientific opinion encourages, nay, compels you to get vaccinated against the disease.

Recovery after COVID-19

If unfortunately you do get infected, you are likely to recover quickly and get your health back, especially if you have been vaccinated. But during the unfolding of the infection and during the process of recovery, there could be lingering health issues, which may prevent you from reaching normalcy. My daughter Indu, during the second wave, had a severe attack, even though she had taken one shot of the vaccine. She has always been an athlete; she runs regularly and plays and coaches tennis. But she took three months to get back her full vigour. During the first few weeks after recovery, her pulse rate was high. Even a small exertion made the pulse shoot up.

She consulted a specialist and he assured her that her lungs were clear and that she would soon get back her full strength. So reassured, and with perseverance, patience and determination, she gradually got her full fitness back and now is as good as ever. So the advice to those of you who are still recovering after a COVID-19 infection is be optimistic. After all, you are rid of the virus. Consult your doctor and get blood tests done, and slowly work your way to fitness. Take small walks, say, for 10 minutes at a time, four or five times a day. Moving about frequently is the medicine for quick recovery. Drink plenty of fluids. Be patient and within a few weeks, you will be as good as gold.

A Healthy Mind

Like the body, the mind also needs nourishment. Drink plenty of water. Get a good night's sleep. These little things ensure a sound mind. Think good thoughts. Listen to music. Visit with family and good friends. These are all balms to ease the wrinkles in the mind. Practise yoga, if you have that bend of mind. It calms your mind, improves your flexibility and has a beneficial effect like that of meditation. Try to avoid the build-up of anxiety. As I experienced first-hand, with just a phrase of encouragement, a psychiatrist can drive away anxiety. Do not nurse such worries. Discuss it with your family members and, if necessary, consult a psychiatrist.

Your Children and Grandchildren

The invitation I offered you in this chapter to join the Fitness Club also extends to your children and your grandchildren, if you have any. You are responsible for the health and welfare of your children. It is the first fifteen years of their life that lay down the bedrock and foundation to live a good life, physically and mentally. I was lucky to have been born in a family that believed in simple, nutritious food, encouraged the pursuit of a variety of interests, spurred us towards liberal thinking and stimulated an appetite for adventure. And that, I suggest, is what you should attempt with your children.

When we were living in Delhi and my children were young, a typical Sunday would start with a trip to Sapru House, in Barakhamba Road, where they used to show children's films. These were thoughtfully produced films to entertain and educate children. We would then visit three libraries, one after the other, where the children would choose their books with great anticipation and excitement. Loaded with books, we would then visit my wife's aunt. While the children would amuse themselves with snacks and banter, my wife and I would socialize with the aunt and her husband. We maintained this Sunday schedule for a year, before I was posted to Moscow, in the Embassy of India.

Winter in Moscow is a great experience. The children would enjoy skating and skiing. Love of sports came naturally to them and this was nurtured by the facilities that nature offered during the Moscow winters. Mina turned out to be a graceful skater, Indu, on return to India, played hockey for Uttar Pradesh in interstate hockey matches, and Param played competitive tennis in the Indian circuit. The tradition has moved on to the next generation.

The grandchildren and great-grandchildren, instead of staring at their cell phones cooped up in a room, go outdoors and play in the open air. For children to develop healthy bodies, it is important that they are exposed to physical activity in the open air.

Children can absorb many things simultaneously. Their brains are eager to absorb anything they come across. Some scientists have estimated that a two-year-old can absorb a million images a day! Introduce your children to knowledge, language skills, music or ideas. Expose the children to ten different things and they will flourish.

Apart from playing competitive tennis at the ITF level, my daughter Indu makes time to coach children below ten years. She has set up a tennis coaching scheme in Sena Vihar, Bangalore, where she lives. Twice a week she engages these children, making them do fitness drills and teaching them tennis skills. Some of the parents of the children who train there have told me that the 1 hour their children spend there is worth a million dollars for them. The children, instead of staring at their cell phones in a cooped-up room, are outdoor, playing in the open air.

I was once invited to the Doon School by the Oxford Blue runner Dev Lahiri, who used to teach there. He asked me to be the chief guest at their annual sports ceremony. I had a special interest in accepting the invitation as Param was then a student there. And Mina and Indu were boarders at the Welham Girls' School in Dehradun.

About a hundred students took part in the 10-kilometre run that day. Through that semester, these boys had run the same distance once a week. So they were well trained and well acclimatized. It was a pleasure to see their enthusiasm and stamina. All schools should be encouraged to have such a curriculum. It can include other outdoor activities apart from running. Children develop healthy bodies through their exposure to physical activity in the open air.

After the Doon School function, I went on to Welham, where a surprise awaited me. It was the school sports day there too. Indira was awarded the rolling trophy for sports and athletics; this, the Principal explained, was for her playing for Uttar Pradesh in the national hockey tournament and for winning the javelin and shot put events in the district sports competition.

The Fun of Maintaining an Exercise Journal

Recently, I opened one of my running journals at random. It was the journal for 1980. I was serving in Kanpur then and was fifty-one years old. One particular page drew my attention. I had written 'Man and child, running as one'. It brought back memories of an early-morning run in a big open field in Chakeri, next to the Air Force campus. Normally there would be no one working out at that time. But that day a young girl, about ten years old, joined the track and started running next to me. I was not running particularly fast, and she easily kept up with my speed. Her father, standing outside the track, was waving and encouraging her to run. We ran two or three laps, more than a kilometre. There was no communication between us except for a brief smile. During those minutes, the man and the child were united in spirit, just rejoicing in the camaraderie of running. A far cry indeed from the anecdotes that I have described in an earlier chapter where the children were mocking me or throwing stones at me!

What Is on Offer When You Accept My Invitation?

So what am I offering when you agree to accept my invitation to a regime of fitness? Well, I am offering to add years to your life and life to your years. The elderly value every extra year, or even month, that they get to live.

In the prime of your health, you may not even think about infirmity and a frail body. But you will be spared such a situation as you advance in age. G.K. Chesterton, the English writer, famously said, 'It is nice to do nothing the whole day, and then relax in the evening.' If you are one of those who like this delightful philosophy, you will end up doing just that, nothing. So get out there, and work your way to lifelong fitness.

ELEVEN

A Peek into My Family and a Final Fitness Round-Up

In this concluding chapter, I would like to deal with two subjects. One, to give you, my readers, a glimpse of my family, which has sustained me. That each member of my family is passionate about the pursuit of fitness is only a small reason for introducing them to you. The main reason is that I am such a happy person because of them. Then I will briefly restate the important message that I want to leave with you regarding fitness.

Why Grandparents Tend to Live Long

There are several studies about the longevity of grandparents. There seems to be a uniformity in the conclusions of these studies. It seems that nature is evolving in such a way that children need their grandfathers and grandmothers because their parents are busy with their work and do not have sufficient time to devote to the children. So the parents recruit their parents for the job. The studies show that evolution works in two ways here. The need for the children to be taken care of and the reduction in stress in grandparents who become caregivers. There is a stipulation that the grandparents should be fit enough to work and play with their grandchildren!

When I was seventy-two years old, I spent a whole year in Washington DC driving Param's two children, Tara and Venkat, six days a week to their tennis coaching centre, 30 kilometres away, and bringing them back safely at the end of the day. They did homeschooling those days and could afford to spend the whole day training to become tennis champions. I have taught all my grandchildren the Tamil language. I have also taught them swimming, cycling, motorcar driving (I had a book published on learning to drive a car) and a chess move or two. I have supervised their learning elements of Carnatic music. They, in turn, have helped me in many ways. Have you ever asked your babies to stand on your back while you are lying down, and made them take a few baby steps? There is no better method to cure you of a backache acquired after a vigorous workout in the gym. It helps if you have a cluster of babies of different weights. You can do research and find the correct baby with the correct weight.

And when they grow up, they run with you on the beach as Shankar did in Pondicherry, and Ashwin, Janu and Akila did in Chennai, or on tracks like Tara and Venkat did.

It is well known that the elderly tend to treat their grandchildren with great affection. Bringing them up is not their direct responsibility and all they need to do is love them and indulge them. At least this is what I have done. So let me briefly describe my family members. But let me say a few words about myself. I was born and brought up in Kozhikode. I did my master's in mathematics from Presidency College, Chennai. My father, V. Parameswara Iyer, practised law in Kozhikode. Wise, with liberal views, he inculcated good values in my sister, Rajam, and me.

In particular, he encouraged me to join the Air Force. He would narrate stories of war heroes who acted bravely in tactical battle situations during the First World War, with no thought for their safety. My mother, Meenakshi, was a housewife and sailed through life spreading love and happiness.

My wife, Kalyani, was full of life and fun, fond of games of all sorts and college tennis champion at Queen Mary's College. She was also the first lady veterinary surgeon in India, graduating from the Madras Veterinary College in 1952. Her father, K. Narayanasami Iyer, was also a lawyer. In addition, he was the undisputed champion of tennis in all of South India in the 1920s. Kay's mother, N. Devanayaki, a pioneering lady, served in the Madras Education Services and retired as inspectress of schools. Kay brought up our three children with love and pride, imparting good values to them. She was my loving companion till she passed away suddenly at the age of eighty. Mina, my eldest, a lawyer and freelance journalist, is the pillar of support to the family. Her well-researched articles focus on the conservation of vital natural resources and fair play towards the downtrodden. One trait that all my children have developed is to pay attention to physical fitness. Mina, though she does not run, has a long and quick stride when she walks. She once took part in a 10-kilometre race in Chennai when she was sixty-two years old. She came third in her age group, overtaking several runners. Anand Ramachandran, her husband, is a distinguished media person for over four decades. He is also a former president of the Advertising Club, Chennai. They have a son, Ashwin, who is married to Kamini Gopalkrishnan. Ashwin and Kamini are in the investment banking industry and live in Bangalore.

Kamini is a manager, regulatory compliance, HSBC. Versatile and artistic, she speaks seven languages and has a melodious singing voice. Ashwin is a senior manager, globalization governance, State Street. He is a born optimist and radiates bonhomie. Fit and fine, Ashwin and Kamini go for long walks in scenic areas, lacing it with occasional jogs.

Indu, my second daughter, is a freelance Russian teacher, interpreter and translator. She runs regularly twice a week and does a 10-kilometre run once a month in about 1 hour. She is also busy these days coaching tennis to young children in our residential society, Sena Vihar, Bangalore. Her husband, Lt Col V. Jayaraman is a retired infantry officer and is an alumnus of Sainik School, Amravathi Nagar, Tamil Nadu, and National Defence Academy. He was the founder-director of Army Welfare Education Services, Pune. Indu has three children. Shankar is the eldest. Like his mother and grandfather, he runs regularly and keeps very fit. He is often mistaken for a college student with his youthful look, though he left college more than a decade and a half ago. During the weekends, he helps out his mother with the tennis coaching classes. An MS in aeronautical engineering from Georgia Tech University, Atlanta, he works with GE (aviation), Bangalore, as a senior engineer (aircraft performance). Shankar is married to Sneha, who is a postgraduate in psychosocial rehabilitation and counselling. She is also fitness-conscious and runs regularly. An artist, Sneha has the gift of converting ordinary things into glorious works of art. She can produce an attractive gift article in no time at all. Their two-year-old girl, Anika, can hang on to a couple of rings with her feet off the ground. It requires tremendous upper body strength to hang like that for several seconds. I, at the other end of the age spectrum, at ninety-two, can do five to six pull-ups on a horizontal bar.

Then comes Akila, Shankar's sister, an architect and an MBA graduate from Indian School of Business. She works as a senior general manager with Godrej Properties, Bangalore. Akila is never short of ideas to break out into new ventures, mostly to do with providing help to the poor and needy. Her husband, Ashwin Nagarajan, an MS in systems engineering from Cornell, US, is a wizard in coding. Their daughter, Vara, has grown into a healthy, bright, smiling and acrobatic baby. Ashwin is also, as you would have guessed by now, an athlete. He runs regularly and is an excellent swimmer too.

Janaki (Janu) arrived next and is the youngest of Indu's three children. She is an Ayurvedic doctor. Fun-loving, she is always the master of ceremonies in family gatherings. She is also fond of games and helps her mother train children in tennis. She is prone to extreme fits of running. Once, a few years ago, she ran for 6 hours without any prior preparation but was none the worse for it. She has also been on a one-week trek to the Nanda Devi in the Himalayas. She is married to Ashwath Ram. A genius in chess, he is a senior business executive and an expert in setting the ambiance for family functions. Ashwath has a bachelor's degree in international business in hotel management from CESAR, Ritz, Switzerland. Ashwath also, needless to say, is a fitness enthusiast. He plays badminton, for 2 hours, almost every day, and is no stranger to our local gym. They have a four-year-old boy Aarav, a handsome fellow with a captivating smile. Being my first great-grandchild, he is special to everyone.

Now I come to my son, Parameswaran. Well, perhaps you have by now gathered that fitness is an obsession in the Iyer family. Param stepped up his fitness regime when he played tennis for St. Stephen's College and Delhi University, and has never stopped running regularly. He joined the Indian Administrative Service in 1981 and has worked both in the government and the World Bank. He served as the Secretary, Drinking Water and Sanitation, in the Government of India from March 2016 to August 2020 when he led the successful implementation of Prime Minister Modi's flagship Swachh Bharat Mission. Param rejoined the government in July 2022, this time as the CEO of NITI Aayog, the national think tank of the government.

Param's wife, Indira, has a doctorate degree in economics. She worked as the Chief Director of Tax Policy Research, Ministry of Finance, in 2017–2020 and is currently a professor of economics at George Washington University, US. She too is a fitness enthusiast and works out regularly. Tara, their eldest, has a doctorate degree in economics from Oxford University, UK, and is an economist at the International Monetary Fund. She played professional tennis, represented India in the Federation Cup and led Duke University, US, to the National Collegiate Athletic Association Division 1 title. She now plays tennis as a hobby but continues her daily fitness and running regime. Venkat, Tara's younger brother, is a postgraduate in environmental science from Columbia University, US, and a senior manager at the World Resources Institute, Washington DC. He too played professional tennis and represented India in the Junior Davis Cup. He captained the Cornell University men's tennis team and led them to the Ivy League title. He is into extreme fitness, and a typical workout for him is a fast-paced 20-kilometre run along the Potomac River, Washington DC, followed by intense strength training in the gym.

A Fitness Round-Up

You Too Can Become Fit, at Any Age

The most important message that I want to leave with you is that, if an ordinary person like me, without any athletic interest or prowess in his youth, could quickly transform himself into a very fit person, and that too when he was approaching the age of fifty, so can any one of you. In my youth, I was interested in chess, bridge and billiards. There is a saying in billiard circles: 'Proficiency in billiards is a sign of a misspent youth'. That was me. I was an unlikely fitness enthusiast. But the transformation happened in just three months. So all you need is three months of regular exercise to become fit. You can choose any form of exercise, so long as your legs are being used – it can be running, walking, cycling, swimming, treadmill, aerobic dancing, anything will do. If you have any doubt about your ability to exercise, consult your doctor and ask for an ECG and a blood test to check that you are free of diabetes. Incidentally, diabetes need not keep you away from exercise. In fact, exercise is good for controlling diabetes, along with diet control and medicines as prescribed by a doctor. Check your kidney function. Do a few of these simple tests, and launch yourself into a fitness regimen. For general good health, as I have mentioned, dental health is crucial. Inadequate dental hygiene can affect your cardiac muscles and your colon. Regular flossing will ensure good dental hygiene.

Till What Age Should One Exercise?

I am sure that you know the answer to this question. Getting fit is not a destination. It is a journey on which you have embarked, a pleasurable, beneficial journey during which you have the stamina and enthusiasm to pursue whatever work or hobby you want to pursue. What exercise gives you is stamina, that is, the capacity to continue doing physical or mental work without getting unduly tired. Speed is inborn but stamina can be developed by anyone by doing aerobic exercises, that is, using your legs. Move about as often as you feel. Even when travelling in an aircraft, stand up and move about the aisle as often as you can. It will prevent fatigue and help in stopping the formation of blood clots in your thighs. Regular aerobic exercise along with strength training will add years to your life. You will appreciate the extra months and years that you will earn. Take my word for it. So do not ask how long you should exercise. It is like asking how long you should continue to eat! Enjoy your new active life and be thankful that you have chosen a colourful lifestyle.

No Visits to Consult a Doctor

Once you enter a phase of life when you are exercising regularly, you won't need to visit a doctor for periodic check-ups. I had fallen into the habit of checking my ECG and even doing a treadmill test before running a marathon or a particularly demanding workout like hill climbing. Once, during one of these tests, the attending senior doctor told me, 'Air Marshal, you don't need to do any medical tests. The very fact that you are running regularly 8 or 10 kilometres is a good indication that you are fully fit.'

Don't Forget to Engage Your Mind

As I have tried to stress in this book, fitness has two dimensions: physical and mental. They have to coexist. You cannot be mentally fit without being physically fit, and vice versa. I have made sure that I keep my mind busy by learning new languages, learning music in my middle age, writing books, playing word games with my family, travelling and reading. These have kept my mind alert.

A Few Words about Eating

Eating is an important part of our lives. Even though I am ninety-two years old, I have not lost my appetite. As a twenty-one-year-old, I was a target of many jokes in the Air Force Academy. My colleagues used to joke that the cadet sitting opposite me at the dining table could not see my face because of the heap of rice on my plate! I have, even today, not lost the zest for eating. The only difference is that my family members no longer joke about it, the reason being that I have not put on any extra weight. I am 5'8" and weigh just 57 kg. I manage this by a combination of the following:

1. A run (though very slow) of at least 2 hours every morning
2. Five gym workouts a week

These activities keep my body's metabolism at a high rate, enabling increased use of calories by the body. I also combine these activities with a wise choice of food. There is nothing special about my food. I eat a wide variety of vegetables. I used to have two whiskies every evening till about a year ago. But, as mentioned in an earlier chapter, I have stopped drinking alcohol. At my age, perhaps, it is not wise to drink alcohol regularly. I don't know whether I will have a drink in the future. If there is a special occasion, who knows.

But I want to reiterate the basics of weight loss or gain. Everyone knows that it is a good thing to reduce weight and get rid of excess fat. Many scientific studies have suggested that obesity is a disease in its own right, and reduced weight is a huge factor in promoting longevity. So here is a tip to reduce your weight.

I have no right to expect all of you to adopt a lifestyle of 2 hours of jogging a day and five workouts in a gym every week. So the next best thing to reduce weight is to eat less. It is as simple as that. It is easy to say 'eat less', but it is extremely difficult to practise it. So here is a tip to reduce your weight, and hold it there.

Some types of food are calorie-dense. Butter, vegetable oils, meat, etc., are calorie-rich. Some other types are calorie-sparse. For example, lettuce and other green leafy vegetables have few calories. You can eat a good portion of these without consuming too many calories. Most vegetables are, in fact, calorie-sparse. So there you have it. Eat plenty of vegetables, including food containing fibre. And try to avoid calorie-dense food. You will find your weight reducing week by week, and month by month. Try it. It works.

Good Wishes and Farewell

With this round-up of fitness tips, I bid you, dear readers, farewell and wish you a long and healthy life in its fullest splendour.

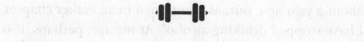

Muscle-Strengthening Exercises

Upper-Body Exercises

Exercise 1: Dumbbell Curls

This exercise strengthens the forearms and biceps. Sit on a stool or on the edge of the bench. Hold one dumbbell in each hand. Start with lighter dumbbells and switch to a heavier dumbbell as you grow in confidence. Let the hands hang down. Raise the arms alternately, your forearms bringing the dumbbells up, till the forearms are vertical. As your right arm goes down to the starting

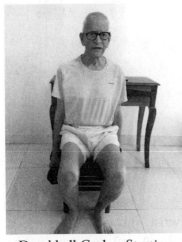 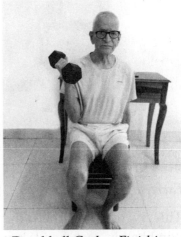

Dumbbell Curls – Starting Position

Dumbbell Curls – Finishing Position (Alternate the Hands)

position, the left arm goes up with the other dumbbell. Do this to a count of 12, then rest for 45 seconds. You have now completed one 'set' of the exercise. Do three such sets, with 45 seconds rest between the sets.

Exercise 2: Sideways Bend

This strengthens the core muscles and the oblique muscles. Stand up, holding a dumbbell in each hand. Bending at your hip, with the knees and elbows straight, bring your left shoulder down as much as possible; then alternatively bring your right shoulder down. Repeat this 12 times. This is one set. Do three such sets, with 45 seconds rest between sets.

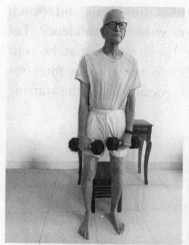 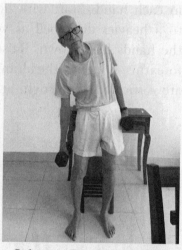

Sideways Bend – Starting Position

Sideways Bend – Finishing Position (Alternate the Arms)

Exercise 3: Wrist Curl

This is to strengthen the wrist muscles. Keeping a dumbbell in each hand, bend down and rest your wrists on your knees. The palms, each holding a dumbbell, should face upwards. Now curl both wrists, upwards. Repeat, as usual, 12 times, and do three sets.

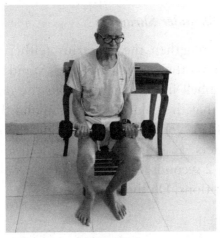

Wrist Curls

Exercise 4: Shoulder Press

This exercise is to strengthen the shoulders and upper back. Sit on a stool. Holding a dumbbell in each hand and looking straight ahead, lift each arm alternately up,

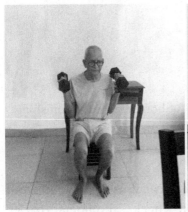 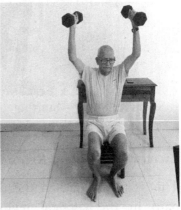

Shoulder Press – Starting   Shoulder Press – Finishing
Position   Position

till the arms are straight and vertical. Repeat 12 times, and do three sets.

Exercise 5: Shoulder Shrug

This is to strengthen the trapezius (either side of the shoulders) and other cervical muscles. Stand straight and hold a dumbbell in each hand. Hold the dumbbells in such a way that the palm is facing you and the knuckles face away from you. Without bending the elbows, lift your shoulders, as far as they can travel, and hold the position for 2 seconds. Slowly bring the shoulders down. Do 12 repetitions. Do three such sets.

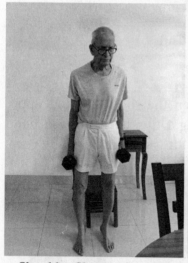 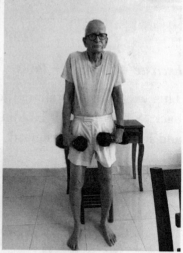

Shoulder Shrug – Starting   Shoulder Shrug – Finishing
         Position   Position

Exercise 6: Shoulder Rotation

This is to strengthen the cervical muscles and prevent pain in the cervical region (neck, shoulders, back). Hold a dumbbell in each hand. Now rotate your shoulders backwards 12 times and forwards 12 times, without bending your elbows. Look straight ahead. This completes one set of shoulder rotations. Do three such sets.

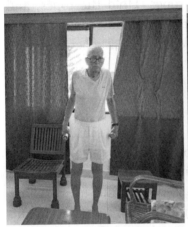 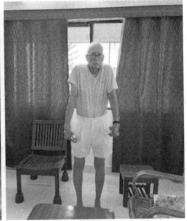

Shoulder Rotation A   Shoulder Rotation B

Exercise 7: Back Exercise

This exercise is to strengthen the back muscles. Use resistance bands for this exercise. Make two sets of ropes by using two bands for each rope. Tie the ropes to two

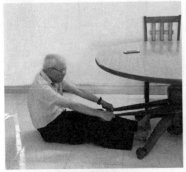 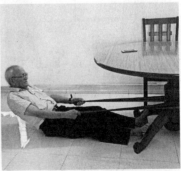

Back Exercise – Starting   Back Exercise – Finishing
Position   Position

fixed points in your room, for example, the legs of a bed or the grill of a door. The idea is to have two sets of flexible ropes that you can pull to exert your back muscles. Sit down on the floor, a comfortable distance away from the anchoring point of the ropes. Hold the ropes, and pull the ropes with your hands, bending your elbows. Keep your back straight and erect. Do 12 repetitions and three sets.

Exercise 8: Bench Press

This exercise is to strengthen the pectoral muscles, which are in your chest region and used for pushing things away from you. Lie down on the exercise bench. If you don't have a bench, a bed will do. Do not use a pillow. Hold a dumbbell in each hand and push your hands up alternately, to a count of 12. Do three such sets.

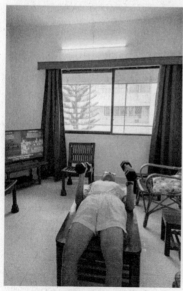 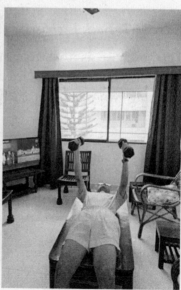

Bench Press – Starting
Position

Bench Press – Finishing
Position

Exercise 9: Bicep Curls

This is to strengthen the biceps. Sit on a stool, holding a dumbbell in each hand. Sit erect and bend both arms simultaneously and hold it for a second, and then come back to the original position. Repeat 12 times and do three sets.

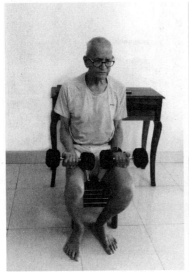 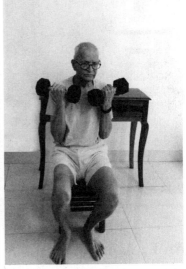

Bicep Curl – Starting Position

Bicep Curl – Finishing Position

Exercise 10: Additional Exercises for the Shoulders

In addition to the above nine exercises, you can devise exercises to work your shoulders through the complete range of their movement. The shoulders are versatile in their capacity to move in different planes, vertical, horizontal and many angles in between. You should use resistance bands to work your shoulders through all these ranges. Anchor two bands at convenient points, hold one band in each hand and work the shoulders by raising your

arms forward, sideways and upwards. Do 12 repetitions
and three sets of each of these exercises.

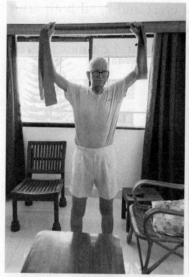 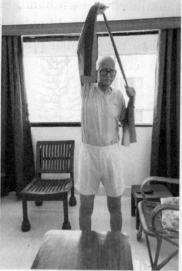

Theraband Shoulder   Theraband Shoulder
Exercise A   Exercise B

An Explanation

This set of exercises strengthens the upper body. It is
not necessary to do all exercises in one session. Choose
four or five of these exercises for one session of your gym
workout. Keep the rest for your next gym session. In this
manner, you will be able to do all the exercises twice a
week. I have deliberately not mentioned the weight of the
dumbbell to be used for each exercise. You should start
with lighter dumbbells and work up to heavier weights,
as you gain confidence and strength. There is no virtue in
trying heavier dumbbells in the beginning; you may get
discouraged and it may cause injury. Progress slowly in
using heavier dumbbells.

Exercises for the Lower Body

So far, we have covered exercises for the upper body, including arms, torso and back. Now we shall go through the exercises required to strengthen the lower body, including the hips and the legs. It is important to keep the legs strong. The legs provide stability for whatever movements we make and, of course, they are crucial for locomotion. Here then are the exercises to be carried out for strengthening them.

Exercise 1: Leg Raise

This exercise is to strengthen the big muscles in front of your thighs. They are a group of four muscles that work as one. They are used to straighten your legs and are used when you walk or run. Tie a pair of weighted ankle straps to the legs. Sit on a stool, with the body erect. Raise each leg alternately, till they are parallel to the ground. Hold the position for 1 second, before

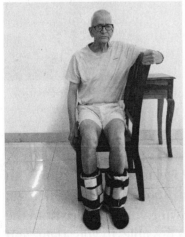 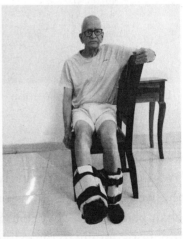

Leg Raise – Starting Position   Leg Raise – Finishing Position
(Alternate the Legs)

bringing each leg down. Do 12 repetitions and do five sets.

Exercise 2: Leg Curls

This is to strengthen the hamstring muscles at the back of your thigh. This set of muscles is responsible for bending your knees and is always used when you walk or run. With the ankle straps still on, stand up and bend your knees alternately, holding the position for a second. Do 12 repetitions and five sets.

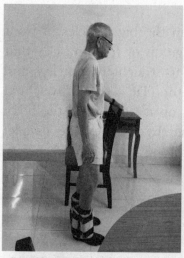 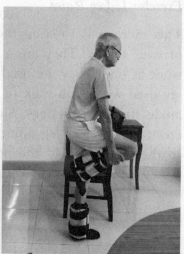

Leg Curl – Starting Position   Leg Curl – Finishing Position
                                              (Alternate the Legs)

Exercise 3: Gluteal Exercises

We use the glutes extensively when we walk or run. With the weighted ankle straps on, stand up erect, holding a chair placed in front of you. Swing your right leg from the hip, horizontally to the extent possible, to your right, and then to the left. Repeat 12 times each. Then turn to your left, and repeat the swings, this time forward and back, 12 times. All the above constitutes one set. Do five such sets. Repeat the exercise with the left leg.

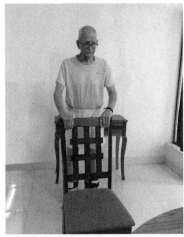

Gluteal Muscles – Starting Position – Horizontal

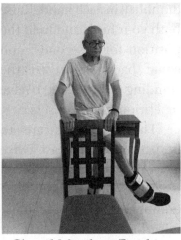

Gluteal Muscles – Finishing Position – Horizontal (Alternate the Legs)

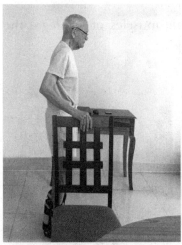

Gluteal Muscles – Starting Position – Vertical

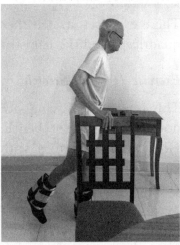

Gluteal Muscles – Finishing Position – Vertical (Alternate the Legs)

Exercise 4: Heel Raise

This exercise strengthens the lower legs. Stand erect with a dumbbell in each hand. Raise both your heels and hold the position for 2 seconds, and come back slowly to the standing position. Do twelve repetitions and five sets.

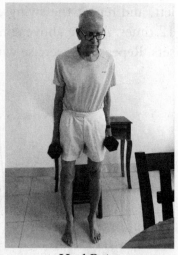

Heel Raise

These exercises are to be performed at least twice a week. The advice given regarding the choice of dumbbells in the previous section holds good for the selection of the ankle straps also. Start with a lighter strap and progress to heavier straps.

Flexibility Exercises

These exercises stretch the big muscles of the leg – the quadriceps and the hamstrings.

Exercise 1: Quad Stretch

This is performed lying face down on a mat or bench. Hold your right toes with your right hand and pull your lower leg back, as much as you can bend; hold this position for a count of 50. Now alternate with the left leg. This is one set. Do three such sets.

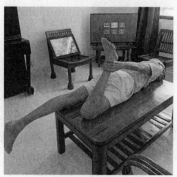

Quad Stretch

Exercise 2: Hamstring Stretch

This is performed standing against a bench or stool 0.5 to 1 metre in height. Stretch your right leg and keep that foot on the stool, without bending the knee. Feel the stretch at the back of your thigh. Hold the position to a count of 50 and return to a standing position. Now alternate with the left leg. This is one set. Do three sets.

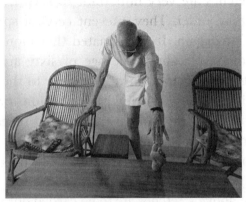

Hamstring Stretch

Exercise 3: Hip Joint

Lie on your stomach on a mat or bench. Raise your upper body as much as you can, and hold this position for a count of 20. Come back to the starting position. This is one set. Do three such sets.

Exercise 4: Shoulder Stretch

Stand erect. Bring your right hand in front of your body with the forehand parallel to the ground. Simultaneously, grip the right shoulder with your left hand and pull it towards the left. Hold the position to a count of 20 and return to the original position. Alternate with the left hand. This is one set. Do three sets. Repeat the exercise, this time holding the right forearm above the head, and pulling the right hand to the left with the left hand. Alternate with the other hand. This is one set. Do three sets.

Exercise 5: Cervical Exercise

These stretches are very important to keep the cervical spine in good order. They prevent cervical spondylosis and associated pain. It is estimated that more than 85 per cent of people above the age of sixty are affected by it. Sitting on a stool, turn your neck to the right, as much as it can turn, and hold the position for a count of 20. Now turn the neck to the left and repeat. Next, turn your head up, as much as possible, and hold for a count of 20. Next, bend your neck down as much as possible and hold for a count of 20.

All the above stretches are to be carried out smoothly and slowly. There should be no jerking or hurried movements.

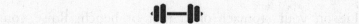

About the Author

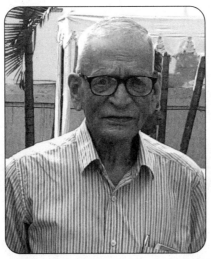

Air Marshal P.V. Iyer, AVSM, VSM (retired), embarked on a fitness journey when he was forty-seven years old. This journey has enabled him to run more than 1,20,000 kilometres. This includes several marathon races of 42 kilometres and an ultra-marathon from Agra to Delhi, a distance of 240 kilometres. Presently, at the age of ninety-two, he continues to run 8 kilometres a day and works out in the gym five days a week.